AIDS, Sexuality and Gender in Africa

The severity of the AIDS epidemic in Africa compels a rethinking of gender relations. *AIDS, Sexuality and Gender in Africa* examines what can be done, particularly by women, to stem the tide of the epidemic. In exploring responses to AIDS in six communities across Tanzania and Zambia, the authors draw lessons which relate more generally to countries throughout the region.

The research on which the book is based examines two hypotheses: first, that the success of strategies to confront the spread of AIDS in Africa rests on the recognition of existing gendered power relations, and second, that AIDS campaigns can be enhanced if built on existing organisational skills and practices, especially amongst women. Individual contributions record the way that AIDS is interpreted within a historical and culturally configured context and review the difficulties and successes of collective activities around AIDS. They show how both men and women must be brought in to the struggle against AIDS, but in ways which entail a re-examination of those inequalities of power which make women vulnerable and at the same time endanger men.

While full recognition is given to the severity of the epidemic and the threat it poses to the population and society, in contrast to some other studies, this account is optimistic in its conclusions. *AIDS, Sexuality and Gender in Africa* will provide a valuable source of information for those wanting to know more about the AIDS epidemic in Africa and the way that gender relations define the issues surrounding the action.

Carolyn Baylies is a Senior Lecturer in the Department of Sociology and Social Policy, University of Leeds and **Janet Bujra** is a Senior Lecturer in the Department of Peace Studies, University of Bradford.

Social Aspects of AIDS

Series Editor: Peter Aggleton
Institute of Education, University of London

AIDS is not simply a concern for scientists, doctors and medical researchers, it has important social dimensions as well. These include individual, cultural and media responses to the epidemic, stigmatisation and discrimination, counselling, care and health promotion. This series of books brings together work from many disciplines including psychology, sociology, cultural and media studies, anthropology, education and history. The titles will be of interest to the general reader, those involved in education and social research, and scientific researchers who want to examine the social aspects of AIDS.

Social Aspects of AIDS
Series Editor: Peter Aggleton
Institute of Education, University of London

AIDS, Sexuality and Gender in Africa

Collective strategies and struggles in Tanzania and Zambia

**Carolyn Baylies and Janet Bujra
with the Gender and AIDS Group**

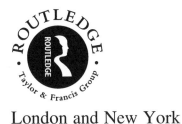

London and New York

First published 2000
by Routledge
11 New Fetter Lane, London EC4P 4EE

Simultaneously published in the USA and Canada
by Routledge
29 West 35th Street, New York, NY 10001

Routledge is an imprint of the Taylor & Francis Group

Typeset in Times by Deerpark Publishing Services Ltd.
Printed and bound in Great Britain by St Edmundsbury Press,
Bury St Edmunds, Suffolk

British Library cataloguing in Publication Data
A catalogue record for this book is available from the British Library

Library of Congress Cataloging in Publication Data
Aids, sexuality and gender in Africa : collective strategies and struggles in Tanzania and
Zambia / Carolyn Baylies and Janet Bujra [editors] ; with the Gender and AIDS Group.
    p. cm. -- (Social aspects of AIDS)
    Includes bibliographical references and index.
    ISBN 1 841 420247 (hc) -- ISBN 1 841 420271 (pbk.)
    1. AIDS (Disease)--Tanzania. 2. AIDS (Disease)--Zambia. I. Baylies, Carolyn L.
(Carolyn Louise), 1947- II. Bujra, Janet M. III. Series.

RA644.A25 A37636 2000
362.1'969792'009678--dc21
                                                                          00-059186
ISBN 1-841-42024-7

Contents

Contributors

Carolyn Baylies has carried out research over many years in Zambia on class, gender, and the political process. She taught briefly at the University of Zambia in the mid 1970s, before joining the University of Leeds in 1980, where she is currently a senior lecturer. As well as teaching sociology, she has been closely involved with the Centre for Development Studies, having served for 6 years as its director.

Janet Bujra has worked as a social anthropologist in both Kenya and Tanzania from the late 1960s, with an extensive record of research on gender, development and class. She taught at the University of Dar es Salaam in the early 1970s and subsequently at the University of Wales, Aberystwyth. She has been a member of staff of the University of Bradford since 1988, where she is currently a senior lecturer in the Department of Peace Studies.

Tashisho Chabala has worked in the AIDS field in Zambia for many years. He trained and practised as a counsellor with Kara Counselling before becoming involved in research. As well as the Gender and AIDS project, he has been involved in work on adolescent perceptions of HIV and girls' education.

Naomi Kaihula has an MA from Dar es Salaam University. Having worked for 30 years as a teacher, she is currently Head of General Studies at Tambaza High School. In addition she does consultancy work as a gender trainer and has conducted research on gender issues in the Mbeya region of Tanzania. She is a member of the Tanzania Gender Networking Programme and Taaluma Women.

Marjorie Mbilinyi is Professor of Education in the Institute of Development Studies, University of Dar es Salaam. She has been involved in several research cum activist projects including co-ordinator of the Rural Food Security Policy and Development group and was a founder member of both the Tanzania Gender Networking Programmes and Women's Research and Documentation Project. She is the author or editor of several books and articles on gender issues in Tanzania.

Faustina Mkandawire holds a diploma in Social Work from the University of Zambia. She has helped with a number of research projects in the fields of health and education in Zambia and was involved with a self help project school in the Lusaka area. She has lived in Trinidad and the UK as well as in Zambia.

Scholastica N. Mokake is a social worker with an Advanced Diploma in Social Work and an MA in International Child Welfare. She has been involved with WAMATA in Dar es Salaam since its origins and has worked as a counsellor, counselling co-ordinator and executive officer for the Dar es Salaam branch of the organisation.

Caroline Shonga holds a Diploma in Social Work from the University of Zambia, as well as a Certificate in Counselling. She participated in a one-year exchange programme for youth leaders and social workers at Ohio State University as well as an international exchange programme for social workers in Finland. She has been involved in a number of HIV/AIDS projects and is a member of the Society for Women and AIDS in Zambia.

Anne Sikwibele is a senior lecturer at the University of Zambia, with a PhD from the University of Illinois, Champaign-Urbana. Her research interests are in social policy issues, with a special focus on gender and development. In 1999 and 2000 she was associated with Oxfam in Zambia as programme co-ordinator for its Education Programme, part of a wider Copperbelt Livelihoods Improvement Programme focusing on interventions to reduce urban poverty.

Series Editor's Preface

The impact of HIV and AIDS on communities all over the world is far from uniform. Most usually, those who are already marginalised and oppressed suffer most, demonstrating the capacity of the virus to exploit the fault lines of an already divided society. In Africa, where the impact of the epidemic has been particularly severe, women have found themselves not only especially vulnerable to infection, but required to shoulder the burden of responsibility for community education and care. This book offers a unique perspective on the challenges that women have faced individually, collectively and as members of community and non-governmental organisations. Drawing on fieldwork conducted in towns and villages in Zambia and Tanzania, it shows how historical and contextual analysis is essential if we are to understand the nature of their response. Using interviews and first hand accounts, it highlights the very real contribution that women make to prevention, education and care. Yet it demonstrates too how prevailing ideologies of masculinity and patriarchy seek to disorient this work, and pose challenges for any effective response. Certain to take its place among the better texts on AIDS and Africa, *AIDS, Sexuality and Gender in Africa* is essential reading for all those working in the fields of development, African studies and health.

Peter Aggleton

Preface

Africa is facing a devastating crisis at the dawn of the twenty-first century, with over 70 per cent of the world's HIV-positive people. Many are struck down at the height of their productive and reproductive years, stretching hard-pressed medical and welfare capacity beyond breaking point, undermining present development efforts, and casting a long shadow over the future. And this in the least developed region of the world, least able to respond effectively to an epidemic of rising deaths and incapacity. Following the wave of decolonisation in the mid-twentieth century, many African countries began to build up the rudimentary welfare systems they had inherited and to improve the living standards of their populations. Death rates began to fall, childhood illnesses were being brought under control and health expectations rose. These positive trends are now being reversed, most appallingly revealed in life expectancy falling in some cases by as many as 25 years against what was otherwise predicted.

Yet the very depth of the crisis entails a liberatory moment, through the collective struggle required if the causes of the epidemic are to be addressed and overturned. Our research, devised within this positive frame, intended to assess how existing strengths could be harnessed toward this task. In practice responses to the epidemic have often been repressive – of youthful sexuality, of women's autonomous capacity to define themselves sexually, of entrepreneurial initiative in the appropriation of sex as a marketable commodity. This brought into question some of our initial optimism.

It is the fate of those who carry out research on the social aspects of AIDS to be overtaken by events and by discursive shifts in the field. If a vaccine or cure had been discovered, then the picture might now look very different (though medical wizardry is not so easily translated into practice). When we began our work, pointing out that AIDS was gendered and that any attempt to halt its progress would require far-reaching transformation in the relations between men and women was still novel. Now such a view is often taken for granted, although more prevalent in official rhetoric than on the ground. We based our work on the proposition that women in Africa had always organised themselves in networks and groups of mutuality and that this organisational capacity meant that women might not only be considered victims but also the authors of their own protection against AIDS. To build on women's existing organisational skills could be a way forward. We stand by this initial thesis, for it has been amply supported in a variety of settings in which we have worked, and in which examples of women's mutuality, creativity, subversiveness and challenge to men's authority are legion.

As the research progressed, however, we recognised the multiple barriers to women's empowerment in the field of sexuality and gender relations. Sometimes we seemed to be doing little more than documenting women's failures to confront men, or their being effectively silenced by men on this topic. It is one thing for women to organise collectively to raise awareness of the dangers of AIDS and its modes of transmission, to raise self-esteem and muster the courage to say no to unwanted sexual contact. It is quite another to challenge men's power in the lonely moment of private relations and to negotiate for safer sex. Unequals cannot negotiate. One can beg and plead whilst the other (at best) may magnanimously concede. This has been a long-standing issue for feminists, enshrined in the 1960s' slogan: 'the personal is political'.

Our research was carried out by a team of scholars (from Britain, Zambia and Tanzania), several of whom were also activists in the AIDS field. The work incorporated a research action element, which carries its own responsibilities. There must be recognition of the dangers of research strategies which expose the most vulnerable to the risk of unprotected abuse or violence in contexts where supportive help is not at hand. Behavioural change, however beneficial, is not achieved overnight. It was our concern, however, to assess how far collective activity around AIDS could itself provide some of the support needed by individuals in pursuing change in their personal relationships.

In recent years, there has been a shift of focus, away from women and towards men as a target group for AIDS interventions. Men's complicity in the spread of AIDS, first flagged by Ankrah (1991) and Obbo (1993), among others, is now stated more starkly: 'the HIV epidemic is driven by men' (Almedal, UNAIDS, quoted in Foreman 1999: viii). Our own work was grounded on the assumption that in any campaign against the spread of HIV infection, men would have to be kept on board. It takes two to make a relationship and women – unless they took a sexually separatist path – needed men to comply with measures of mutual protection if they were to save themselves.

What is important is *men's* increasing recognition of their role as vectors of infection, given their greater geographic and social mobility and their power to control women's lives and bodies (see Agenda 1998; Foreman 1999). While continuing to focus on and support the more vulnerable (women, the young), it is increasingly seen as essential to face down the powerful, taking note of the opportune nature of such a challenge at a point where men are also vulnerable, when casual unprotected sex as an assertion of masculinity is in practice a death wish and lack of protection within marriage can bring mutual demise. The challenge is to devise interventions which, whilst recognising gender inequity, essentialise neither 'men' nor 'women'. Masculinity comes in many guises.

It is our contention that the threat of AIDS has added a new dimension to gender relations in a context where the predominant mode of transmission is through heterosexual contact. Many continue to deny or resist 'seeing' its implications for gender relations, but some men are beginning to realise that AIDS renders women a lethal threat to them and their carefully tended structures of patriarchal control (still heavy in most parts of Africa). Both men and women see their lives in danger from 'normal sexual relations', but if the 'solution' is greater mutuality and equality within intimate relations, this necessarily threatens men's power to define sexual practice and even their ability to father children and further their line.

One facet of the AIDS crisis which did not become apparent until we were well into our programme of research was the ambivalence, and sometimes the fear and hatred, that older people have for the young. AIDS epitomised the tragic havoc that unruly young people might wreak, and it was common for them to be blamed for the epidemic. Far from a solidarity of purpose amongst women, there were contradictory currents of jealous bitterness expressed by (some) older women towards the younger generation, mingled with terror and concern, especially when the young people were their sons and daughters. Attempts to facilitate the empowerment and protection of young women reflected genuine concern and compassion, but could also be transformed into bids to repress and control them more effectively.

Our research was conceived as an analytical, although also an involved and committed, investigation of women's efforts to protect themselves from the devastation of AIDS. But AIDS, shocking as its destructive outcomes have been, cannot be isolated from the web of problems which many face. It has spread through the fabric of other difficulties in people's lives – impoverishment, migration to towns, selling sex in order to eat, gendered and generational inequities. It follows that the effectiveness of AIDS interventions may be limited if single-stranded or merely health-focused. They need to be embedded in a broader struggle for solutions to people's straightened circumstances, to take on board poverty through income generation projects, ignorance through literacy campaigns, social injustice through political organisation, religious bigotry through bridge building between different faiths and so on.

Here, AIDS work faces the same hurdles as any other development initiative: apathy, extra stress and pressure on limited resources of time or money, projects which can be hi-jacked by the already well-placed, bids for personal as well as collective improvement, corruption, abuse and manipulation of external contacts, the use of the most vulnerable to promote careers and so on. In the course of these 'development' struggles, the focus on AIDS work is often blurred or lost. But there are also more positive examples, providing insight on how, while meeting immediate objectives and supporting members, interventions can expose those aspects of gender relations which drive the epidemic and can contribute toward their transformation.

This book is about the chequered attempts to deal with the threat of AIDS in two severely affected countries in Africa: Tanzania and Zambia. In particular it looks at how the epidemic and responses to it have impacted on gender relations. It documents how the best laid plans of governments, activists, ordinary people and researchers face contradictions and set-backs. It also illustrates the tremendous courage and fortitude of those who go on trying, and it is to them that we dedicate our work.

Acknowledgements

This book is the product of the commitment and labour of two research teams in Zambia and Tanzania, whose individual and collective efforts were crucial to its fruition. Personal circumstances, heavy workloads and distant assignments prevented some members being involved in the final analysis and writing of the text, but the contribution of all must be fully acknowledged. Particular mention should be made of the work of Beatrice Liatto-Katundu and Marjorie Mbilinyi, who served as local co-ordinators of the research teams in Zambia and Tanzania. Alongside full-time work as executive officers of large NGOs in their respective countries, each managed budgets, conducted team meetings, and, most importantly, organised the workshops which set the research in motion (Beatrice in Lusaka in 1994) and officially wound it up (Marjorie in Dar es Salaam in 1996). In bringing together a range of AIDS activists and researchers, these were crucial to the development of initial objectives and working procedures and to ensuring local dissemination of findings.

Several others who were part of the project from its beginning must also be mentioned. Lillian Mushota, a lawyer by profession, and committed for many years to ensuring that women's legal rights are protected, not least in widowhood, was instrumental in conducting an overview of AIDS activities in Luapula Province and beginning the work in Mansa. Olive Munjanja, finding time from her work as executive officer of the Zambian Association for Research and Development, laid the groundwork for the research in Kanyama, carrying out initial key informant interviews and later facilitating focus group discussions. Zubaida Tumbo-Masaba, a Senior Research Fellow with the Institute of Kiswahili Research at the University of Dar es Salaam and a founding member of the Women's Research and Documentation Project, brought to bear a research background in adolescent sexuality in co-ordinating the work in Dar es Salaam. Feddy Mwanga, as Secretary General of the Tanzanian branch of Society of Women and AIDS in Tanzania, conducted research in the vicinity of Tanzania's capital, with a focus on Tegeta Village in Kinondoni District. Working in Dar itself were two young activists, Japhet Lutimba and Julius Mwabuki, who brought enormous enthusiasm and dedication to the task. As members of WAMATA Youth, their participation ensured that the research took on board issues of generation as well as gender.

Those who appear as authors of chapters in this book comprised additional members of the teams – Tashisho Chabala, Faustina Mkandawire, Caroline Shonga, Anne Sikwibele and Carolyn Baylies in Zambia and Scholastica Mokake, Naomi Kaihula and Janet Bujra in Tanzania. But these do not exhaust the number of those involved in the project, for others worked as research assistants or associates. Appreciation needs to be extended to the contribution of Mrs Wakalala, Elizabeth Mukwita, Miriam Mundia, M. Sifuniso, and Kapenda Kapenda in Kapulanga; David Mwaipopo in Rungwe; Augustine Mkandawire and John Zulu in Kanyama; Haji Ayoub Mtangi and Helena Anthony in Lushoto; Agnes Lusesa in Dar es Salaam; and Arnold Kunda and Anastasia Mwewa in Mansa. An enormous debt of gratitude is extended to them all.

Abbreviations

AIDS	Acquired immune deficiency syndrome
AIDSCOM	US AIDS NGO, Tanzania
AMREF	African Medical Research Foundation
CCM	*Chama cha Mapinduzi* (The Revolutionary Party, Tanzania)
CHEP	Copperbelt Health Education Project
DANIDA	Danish Government Aid Agency
EU	European Union
GPA	Global Programme on AIDS
HIV	Human immunodeficiency virus
HIVOS	Humanistic Institute for International Cooperation, Holland
HNWC	Health Neighbourhood Watch Committee
ICASA	International Conference on AIDS and STDs in Africa
IEC	Information, Education and Communication programmes
IFI	International Financial Institution
KABP	Knowledge, Attitudes, Beliefs and Practices
MS	Danish Association for International Co-operation
NACP	National AIDS Control Programme (Tanzania)
NASTLP	National AIDS/STD/Tuberculosis and Leprosy Programme (Zambia)
NGO	Non-governmental organisation
NORAD	Norwegian Aid Agency
ODA	Overseas Development Agency (UK)
PUSH	Peri-urban Self Help
RDC	Residents' development committee
SAT	Southern Africa Training programme
SATF	Social Action Trust Fund
SDA	Seventh Day Adventist Church
SHD	Sustainable Human Development
SHDEPHA	Service, Health and Development for People living with HIV/AIDS, Tanzania
STDs	Sexually Transmitted Diseases
SWAAT	Society for Women and AIDS in Tanzania
SWAAZ	Society for Women and AIDS in Zambia

TAMWA	Tanzania Media Women's Association
TAP	Tanzania AIDS Project
TASO	The AIDS Organisation (Uganda)
TBA	Traditional birth attendant
TDH	Terre des Hommes (Switzerland)
TGNP	Tanzania Gender Networking Programme
UCZ	United Church of Zambia
UN	United Nations
UNAIDS	Joint United Nations Programme on HIV/AIDS
UNDP	United Nations Development Programme
UNICEF	United Nations Children's and Education Fund
USAID	United States Agency for International Development
UMATI	The Tanzania Family Planning Association
UWT	*Umoja wa Wanawake Tanzania* (the Tanzania National Women's Association)
WAMATA	*Walio katika Mapambano ya AIDS, Tanzania* (Those in the struggle against AIDS in Tanzania)
WHO	World Health Organisation
WILDAF	Women in Law and Development in Africa
YWCA	Young Women's Christian Association
ZARD	Zambia Association for Research and Development
ZNAN	Zambia National AIDS Network

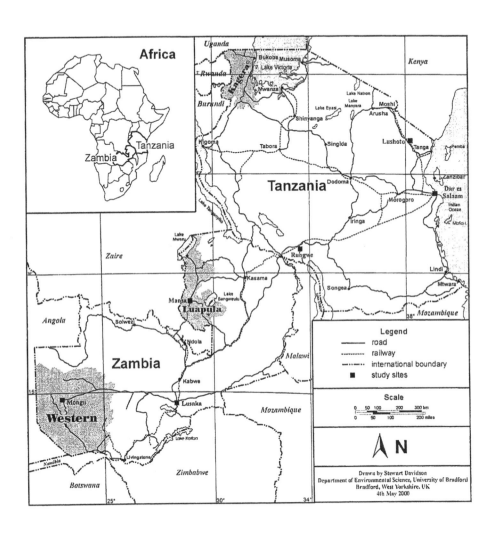

1 Perspectives on gender and AIDS in Africa

Carolyn Baylies

Introduction

For those countries worst affected, AIDS represents a human tragedy and developmental emergency of huge proportions. Yet by exposing how prevailing gender relations and other patterns of structured inequality are implicated in its spread, the AIDS pandemic offers the possibility of change – indeed necessitates it. It lays bare the need to engage with the mutuality of interests among sexual partners in seeking forms of protection which can ensure survival of themselves, their children and their communities.

Our focus on the potential for harnessing women's organisational capacities around campaigns of protection and support highlights contradictions which the pandemic poses. Women are a source of strength and the backbone of both public sector and community-based initiatives aimed at care and protection (Whelan, 1999). In investigating how the energy, expertise and traditions of mutual support among women can contribute to the struggle against AIDS, we have drawn on Ulin's observation that:

> The solidarity of women in rural African communities may be their greatest source of strength for coping with the AIDS epidemic...
>
> (Ulin, 1992: 64)

However, AIDS also exposes women's vulnerability. Both men and women are affected by AIDS, but women particularly so, given how gender relations configure with sexual behaviour and economic security. Gender relations not only underlie women's particular vulnerability; they also inhibit women's attempts to protect themselves and their families. If interventions around AIDS are to be effective, they must address the factors which drive the epidemic. Such factors are deep-seated and intransigent, embedded in the very power relations which define male and female roles and positions, both in intimate relations or the wider society. Women (and men) need protection *now* and cannot wait for deep structural changes. However, we argue that it is crucial for short term interventions to be consistent with and not contradict more long term objectives, so that they contribute to rather than inadvertently reinforce those power relations which drive the epidemic. The question is how far women's organisations can contribute to the struggle against AIDS along these lines.

Keeping in mind the assumption that strategies must address underlying causes, we explore factors of vulnerability as a preliminary to reviewing strategies of intervention. We review shifts in discourse from women being first 'hidden', then blameworthy, and then seen as occupants of marginalised positions, noting the way in which vulnerability is configured through gender relations in both public and private spheres, and varies for women (and men) in accord with age, marital situation and other factors. We then turn to strategies of protection, noting shifts in discourse and practice towards an increased acknowledgement of social context and the incorporation of local knowledge and experience. The difficulties of devising strategies which effectively link short and long term objectives are explored. Finally, we examine the specific potential of women's collective efforts at community level in campaigns of protection against HIV, with reference to limitations and pitfalls as well as strengths.

The Joint United Nation's Programme on HIV/AIDS' (UNAIDS) charts the AIDS epidemic globally. It documents its scale and severity in Africa and the way in which that continent's population has disproportionately borne its brunt. Overall, by the end of 1999 it was estimated that 24.5 million people were living with HIV/AIDS on the African continent (UNAIDS, 2000b). The pattern of affliction varies, with those countries in eastern and southern Africa most affected (UNAIDS, 2000c).[1] However, the overall rate of adult prevalence for the continent, at an estimated 8 per cent, is far, far higher than that of any other region of the globe, the next closest being the Caribbean at 1.96 per cent (UNAIDS, 1999g).

That AIDS has gained so tight a grip on a number of African countries is partly a consequence of their poverty (Ankrah, 1991; Panos, 1992; Schoepf, 1997; Cohen, 1998b), as represented by deficiencies in nutrition, hazards of living, and lack of access to medical care. In some cases, national indebtedness and regimes of structural adjustment have exacerbated difficulties of securing livelihoods and restricted access to health services, further contributing to a broad risk ecology in respect of AIDS (Ankrah, 1991, 1996; Sanders and Sambo, 1991; Cohen, 1998c). The very character of the (distorted) development they have experienced has figured in the spread and entrenchment of HIV/AIDS in these countries. Through its impact on productivity and the costs it entails, the epidemic is operating in turn to frustrate further developmental progress, so much so that it has been belatedly acknowledged by international institutions to be the foremost development issue for the present and foreseeable future (Madavo, 1999; World Bank, 1999).

However, the grip which AIDS has in Africa is also a consequence of the pace of social change, as registered in high rates of mobility in search of economic security, later marriage in consequence of more widespread education, a loosening of former mechanisms of sex education and, in consequence, changing patterns of sexual behaviour. Setel (1996: 1169) argues, for example, that in the Kilimanjaro region of Tanzania, AIDS has been perceived by many as being bound up with a 'slowly emerging cultural crisis – a crisis rooted in transformations that began before the turn of the century'. Ideas about sex and work – reproduction and production – have been fashioned in accord with changing opportunities and new discourses, particularly in the lives of youth, who, in seizing upon them and apparently discarding behaviours and practices which were formerly valued, have been both vilified and placed in positions of greater vulnerability in respect of AIDS. Their elders in turn have seen youths' susceptibility to HIV as vindication of their own anxiety about the apparent abandonment of those former customs which had provided the social cement for the community's very survival. In this sense, AIDS has generated a similar unease with changing norms of sexual behaviour – albeit attached to different specific practices – as occurred in the North.

Gender relations as key to an understanding of the AIDS epidemic

All are potentially susceptible to AIDS. HIV crosses all lines of social division. At the same time social circumstances may entail particular vulnerability. Gender relations serve in this regard as an important component of the way AIDS has impacted on African societies. While there is a substantial problem of parent to child transmission in many countries, and some transmission via blood and between gay men, by the far the most significant mode of transmission is through heterosexual encounters. Relative proportions of adult males and females infected vary from place to place, but UNAIDS has estimated that by the end of the century, twelve or thirteen women were being infected in Africa for every ten men (UNAIDS, 1999g). Partly because those infected at an earlier age may live longer with HIV, there may be increasing disparity in prevalence rates for males and females. However, differentials also reflect disproportionate risk to women. In Ndola, on Zambia's Copperbelt, for example, adult prevalence was 32 per cent for females as against 23 per cent for males in the late 1990s and in Kisumu, Kenya, respectively, 30 and 20 per cent (UNAIDS, 1999c). In accounting for these patterns, it is essential to understand both how gender relations create vulnerabilities and the specific way the epidemic has impacted on women.

Early on in the epidemic, the experience of men served to define the range of presenting symptoms and the course of the illness (Bury, 1991; Sherr, 1996), so that women disappeared, indeed were not even in the picture (Patton, 1993). If the early association of HIV, not just with homosexuality, but also with the use of injecting drug use, led to a delay in the recognition of a new illness condition by medics in Africa (Mukonde, 1992), it also led to a delayed understanding of its impact on women. But even when women were taken into account, it was typically via discourses of blame. They have characteristically been viewed as responsible for transmitting the virus, whether as prostitutes infecting their clients or mothers infecting their children, along lines characterised by Patton (1993) of women being treated variously as vaginas or uteruses, by Carovano (1991) as whores or mothers and, more gently by Sherr (1993) as vectors or vessels.

Blame is most consistently and strenuously attached to those women regarded as responsible for the rapid spread of AIDS in Africa in their capacity as sex workers (de Bruyn, 1992; Schoepf, 1993b). But a broad brush of disapproval has often been extended to women in general as being responsible for AIDS, as indicated by Obbo's analysis of children's essays in Uganda (as reported in Barnett and Blaikie, 1992) and associations drawn between AIDS and traditional illnesses with similar symptoms, which have been characteristically attributed to women's 'polluting influence' on the men having sex with them in particular circumstances.[2] Also, in Africa as elsewhere, it is women who are blamed for the birth of a child with HIV, as 'contaminated vessels bearing condemned babies' in the words of Bassett and Mhloyi (1991: 146).

A number of writers (Ankrah, 1991; Bassett and Mhloyi, 1991; Carovano, 1991; Hamlin and Reid, 1991; Schoepf *et al.*, 1991; de Bruyn, 1992; Schoepf, 1992, 1993a,b; Ulin, 1992; Berer and Ray, 1993; Obbo, 1993; Doyal, 1994; Sherr, 1996, among others) have eloquently and forcefully made the case for bringing women into the picture as regards HIV/AIDS, particularly where heterosexual transmission predominates, not as blameworthy but as inhabiting a context in which they are often highly vulnerable to infection. In recognition of the increasing number of women affected and the way the burden of care falls on women's shoulders at both family and community level, Peter Piot (1998) Executive Director of UNAIDS, has acknowledged AIDS to be a 'woman's epidemic'.[3] However, if women have thus come onto AIDS agendas, it has arguably been to a lesser degree than need implies (Long, 1996). As Farmer (1999) stresses, many women with HIV lack support and continue to be effectively silenced, not least by virtue of the marginalisation which increases their probability of being infected.

But important shifts *have* occurred in discourses around women and AIDS during the course of the epidemic's history. Under the auspices of the Global Programme on AIDS (GPA), and later UNAIDS, initial concern to counter discrimination against those with AIDS has been transformed into a more comprehensive human rights approach (Mann *et al.*, 1992; Seidel, 1993; Mann and Tarantola, 1996; UN, 1996) which posits that the very marginalisation of particular groups, as materialised in their lack of rights and the inequalities describing their situation, has restricted their ability to protect themselves. By insisting that women's rights are necessarily *human* rights and at least in theory universally applicable, then particular factors, be they cultural conventions or structural inequality, can be cited as obstacles to protection requiring attention within a global, moral framework.

Factors of vulnerability

Women's vulnerability to AIDS follows from social, but also physiological factors. All else being equal, the probability of male to female transmission is estimated to be two to four times that of female to male transmission (UNAIDS, 1997). The reasons are higher concentrations of HIV in semen than in vaginal fluid, a larger area of exposed female than male genital surface area, greater permeability of the mucous membranes of the vagina compared with those of the penis, and longer period of exposure of semen within the vaginal tract (Doyal, 1994; WHO, 1995; Baden and Wach, 1998). Untreated sexually treated diseases (STDs) can increase the probability of HIV transmission in both men and women by as much as ten times (McNamara, 1991; Parker and Patterson, 1996; UNAIDS, 1997). However, because STDs in women are often asymtomatic, they are less likely to be treated. Behavioural factors complicate the situation, with women typically having poorer access to STD care because of distance, costs, adequacy of facilities and the way the stigmatising nature of the condition deters them from seeking formal assistance.

Increasing attention has been given to the significance of genital ulcer disease (chancroid) (Doyal, 1994), which is particularly common in some African contexts (Pitts *et al.*, 1995; Ballard, 1999) and strongly associated with increased risk of HIV infection (UNAIDS, 1999c). In addition, repeated infections of gonorrhoea, chlamydia and other reproductive tract infections, through their association with infertility (McNamara, 1991), can sometimes lead women toward greater sexual activity in an attempt to conceive, or, in contributing to the forced ending of marriage, can result in women being placed at increased risk of HIV (de Bruyn, 1992). HIV itself has a direct impact in reducing fertility (Carpenter *et al.*, 1997; du Lou *et al.*, 1999; Gregson *et al.*, 1999). When a woman who is already infected becomes pregnant, however, the progression of HIV may be accelerated and complications of pregnancy and delivery increased (Berer, 1999; Gregson *et al.*, 1999).

While physiological factors increase the risk of transmission to women from unprotected sex and accelerate the course of illness in a woman who is living with HIV, women's social location can also place them in the context of risk or inhibit their ability to protect themselves. As Heise and Elias (1995: 931) note, 'in large measure, women's vulnerability to HIV infection derives from their low status in society'. Similarly, Ankrah (1991) describes women as a 'subordinate sector', in referring to their low status and powerlessness in connection with AIDS. Powerlessness is a frequent theme. For Hamlin and Reid (1991: 3) it is precisely the link between powerlessness and risk of HIV which is 'the key to understanding the sources of women's vulnerability'. Bassett and Mhloyi (1991) refer to women's limited control to determine their own lives, Rivers and Aggleton (1999) to their lesser ability (than men) to control the nature and timing of sexual activity and Ulin (1992) to their frequent inability to negotiate change in sexual behaviour. The context, content and nature (or specificity) of such powerlessness varies, alternatively describing either a general failure in women's capacity to secure their needs or their specific inability to ensure protection within sexual encounters.

It is precisely the *link* between control over potentially risky sexual relations and women's position within the wider society that is crucial, however, for an understanding of vulnerability and the way in which HIV moves through a population. Heise and Elias (1995: 939) allude to the two poles of this relationship when commenting that 'women often have too little power within their relationships to insist on condom use, and they have too little power outside of these relationships to abandon partnerships that put them at risk'. Understanding this relationship requires a preliminary examination, on the one hand, of gender relations within the public sphere which determine women's ability to realise capabilities and attain a 'good life' and, on the other, power and control in intimate social systems (Ahlemeyer and Ludwig, 1997).

Gender relations of inequality within the public sphere

The United Nations Development Programme's (UNDP) gender related development index (UNDP, 1995), which provides a rough approximation of women's social position on a country by country basis, reveals that women's capability to enjoy a 'good life' consistently falls short of men's.[4] Women live longer than men, but do less well overall with respect to other capabilities. Elson (1995) has argued that to the extent that there is systematic disadvantage to women across a range of capabilities – being well-nourished, enjoying good health and long lives, and being able to read and write, participate freely in the public sphere, have time to oneself and enjoy dignity and self esteem – there is male bias in development outcomes. Such bias, residing both in the 'deep structures' of society and reflected in day to day behaviour, is embedded in legislation, official policy and practice, political and religious ideologies, and cultural conventions.

Individually and collectively these factors bear on women's vulnerability to HIV (WHO, 1995; UNAIDS, 1997; UNAIDS, 1998b, 1999d). In African countries, women's lesser access to education and lower levels of literacy contribute to their more limited access to information about STDs and HIV (de Bruyn, 1992; UNAIDS, 1997). Their poorer access to health care, and particularly to appropriate health care, mean that their illnesses are often treated less quickly and less adequately (de Bruyn, 1992). They may be subject to legal stipulations which limit their access to or the continuity of economic resources and place them in positions of dependence on men, as fathers, brothers or husbands (WHO, 1995). In many countries, women are still legal minors or only recently recipients of full adult status in the eyes of the law (Akeroyd, 1997). The cultural conventions which guide their socialisation – sometimes reinforced by religious ideologies – may inhibit them from asserting themselves in public arenas and thereby adding their voices to the process of policy formulation. Differences in capabilities necessarily vary from place to place and for women in different social locations within a given society. Collectively, and however specifically defined, they are a reflection of gender relations.

They are perhaps most importantly coalesced in material conditions. While women contribute more hours of labour than do men (UNDP, 1995), they have less access to income and possess much less wealth. Women's economic position, often involving a greater or lesser dependence on men, is a consequence of the way the kind of work men and women do articulates with valuation of labour. To the extent that much of their labour characteristically does not command market value, because confined to the domestic sphere, women become dependent on those members of their household or kin group who operate in the cash economy. Where opportunities to gain marketable skills and education are restricted for women, their possibility for combining non-market with market valued activities is reduced.

Such dependence is often expressed – both within and outside marriage – through sexual relations. Indeed sex has been referred to as the currency by which women and girls are frequently 'expected to pay for life's opportunities, from a passing grade in school to a trading license or permission to cross a border' (UNAIDS, 1997: 4). Akeroyd (1997) therefore emphasises the importance of seeing the sexual act as bound up not just with personal relations of intimacy but also with economic strategies. In practice, this may take many different forms, not easily captured by such concepts as prostitution, monogamy or multiple partners (Heise and Elias, 1995). The specific way in which economic dependence figures in sexual relations affects the extent to which women are able to exert control, and in particular, to ensure protection against HIV. In a significant and profound way it brings the broader situation of women (informed by the nature of gender relations within the public sphere) into the private sphere.

Gendered power in the context of intimate relations

Relations of intimacy are informed by the same cultural prescriptions and notions of personhood that operate within the larger society to influence the gender division of labour, educational opportunities, the legal system and the gendered structure of employment. Thus 'outcomes' or manifestations of gender ideologies can be seen in both the wider society and in intimate social systems and mutually reinforce one another. However, they manifest themselves in specific ways, taking form as sexual practices and sexual understandings within the sphere of private relations.

These often involve a prescription of relative passivity for females, and the according of sexual decision making and initiative to men, along with a tolerance of men's greater sexual mobility both prior to and after marriage. Women for their part are often expected to give but not receive pleasure. While such prescriptions and assumptions necessarily vary among cultures and within a given society in accord with specific social location, there are commonalities in the gendered power relations across many circumstances (Rivers and Aggleton, 1999; Rweyemamu, 1999). Socialisation into sexual matters, including the language used, and the way sex is approached, understood and valued, often varies as between males and young females. In consequence, women may be at considerable disadvantage in being able to exert equal influence over the nature and meaning of sexual encounters (Holland *et al.*, 1998).

The terms of such 'negotiation' necessarily vary with the specific circumstances of the sexual actors involved and the nature of the sexual encounter. Ahlemeyer and Ludwig (1997) draw attention to different types of intimate social systems – romantic, hedonistic, matrimonial and prostitutive – whose dynamics may differ fundamentally from one another, not least as regards perception of AIDS-related risks and the possibility for enacting preventive measures. This characterisation resonates with Carovano's (1995) depiction of variability in the meaning of sexual encounters across a number of dimensions:

> Men and women engage in sexual relations for an array of reasons that range from the pursuit of pleasure, desire for intimacy, expression of love definition of self, procreation, domination, violence or any combination of the above, as well as others. How people relate sexually may be linked to self-esteem, self-respect, respect for others, hope, joy and pain. In different contexts, sex is viewed as a commodity, a right or a biological imperative; it is clearly not determined fully by rational decision-making.
>
> (Carovano, 1995: 3,4)

Women's ability to negotiate may be greater in casual encounters or in more straightforwardly commercial transactions than within 'trust' relationships, and particularly in marriage. However, whether in transactional sex or in romantic or matrimonial relationships, any transgression of power relations may make protection difficult.

Negotiation is not even at issue in those sexual encounters characterised by coercion or violence. Coercion may be an element in all relations involving economic dependence, but overt violence is also a feature of many sexual relationships and a particular matter of concern where HIV prevalence is high (Baden and Wach, 1998; Gordon and Crehan, 1999). While applying within marriage, it is also characteristic of many relationships among adolescents (Wood *et al.*, 1998; Jewkes, 1999). Rape is also a matter of deep concern, both in situations of political conflict and social dislocation (Turshen and Twagiramariya, 1998) and in more 'normal' circumstances. Its pervasiveness – and the seriousness of the accompanying threat of HIV infection – is grotesquely highlighted in South Africa, where insurance has come onto the market to cover medical costs for women infected by the virus in this way (gender-aids@hivnet.ch 15.10.99).

Gender as incorporating men

Shifts from the discourse of blame to one of vulnerability and human rights
have increasingly entailed the description of women's situation in terms of
gender relations. Increasingly this gender perspective is taken up not just as a
means of exploring the implications of gendered power relations and gender
ideologies for women, but also the way in which *men* are specifically endan-
gered by ideologies of masculinity. In the early 1990s, Ankrah (1991: 972)
pointed to the need for reassessing the concept of maleness and argued for
male empowerment, so that men might be 'intellectually and emotionally
released from the cultural entrapments that require the female to be submis-
sive'. Heise and Elias (1995) remarked that empowering women necessarily
requires a redefinition of what it means to be male, de Bruyn (1992) called for
further research into concepts of virility and male family concerns, and Obbo
(1993) drew attention to the need for a change in the behaviour and attitudes
of men and boys. There has thus been recurrent insistence that an analysis of
gender relations requires full understanding of the knowledge, motivation and
constraints faced by both men and women, precisely because it is the *relationship* between men's volition and women's dependence and restricted agency
which are at issue.

Gender relations have been increasingly brought to the fore in the work of
international agencies, as has a specific concern with the harmful effects of
masculine ideologies. The work of Reid (n.d.) and others, under the auspices
of UNDP, has been of considerable importance in registering a transition,
marked by the Cairo Conference on Population and Development in 1994, to
a new analytical framework which locates the interlinkages of 'human sexuality, desires and pleasures, women's health and empowerment' with 'men's
engagement' within a broader political and cultural context. Specific attention
to men's engagement and positioning in regard to heterosexual transmission
of HIV has also been directly addressed by Carovano (1995) and more
recently by Rivers and Aggleton (1998) and Bujra (2000c). However, there
is need for more work in this area. As Whelan's (1999) review of publications
and practice in respect of gender and AIDS suggests, there remains a substantial lapse in understanding about male sexuality and the social and economic
forces which sustain it.

Social divisions: facing the epidemic from different social locations

Neither women nor men constitute a homogeneous category and patterns of
vulnerability must be assessed along other lines also. Most important among
them are age, class and marital status.

The particular vulnerability of young people

In most African countries it is men and women in the midst of their productive and reproductive lives who are most likely to become infected by HIV and to die. However, given a typical age difference between partners of five to ten years, females tend to be infected at a younger age. UNAIDS' study of four urban areas in Africa in the late 1990s, for example, found 3 and 4 per cent of males aged 15–19 infected in Kisumu, Kenya, and Ndola, Zambia, respectively, as against 23 and 15 per cent of females (UNAIDS, 1999c).

On a global basis, half of all new HIV infections involve those in the 15–24 age group (UNAIDS, 1999g). Younger women are especially vulnerable (Reid and Bailey, 1992; UNAIDS, 1998a), in part, it is believed, because of the immaturity of their cervix (WHO, 1995; Baden and Wach 1998) and vulnerability to non-consensual sex. Young women are also particularly susceptible to STDs which increase the risk of HIV transmission. The four city comparative study (UNAIDS, 1999c), for example, found that almost half of females aged 15–19 in the two cities with highest HIV prevalence had been exposed to the virus which causes herpes. Chlamydial infection was also more common in the younger age groups, particularly among women.

Young people often have limited information about reproductive and sexual health generally as well as about STDs and HIV. Health services are seldom designed for their needs (Fuglesang, 1997; Rivers and Aggleton 1999). In many cases services catering for sexual health are located in family planning or STD clinics, neither of which adolescents may feel comfortable in approaching (Webb, 1997a). Lack of information and socialisation, which encourages bravado on the part of males while discouraging both the acquisition and articulation of sexual knowledge on the part of young women, may also be factors which place young people at a disadvantage in protecting themselves from HIV (Rivers and Aggleton, 1999).

In many parts of Africa, 'traditional' forms of sex education delivered through initiation ceremonies or by older family members have lost their importance (Ntukula, 1994), and structured means of imparting knowledge to young people are much less common than formerly. At the same time, there are often strong sanctions against open discussion of sexual matters across adjacent generations. Nor have schools adequately taken up the task, although in some cases programmes are being introduced. In consequence, young people frequently learn about sex from their peers, and not always accurately (Baylies and Bujra *et al.*, 1999).

It is important, however, not to underestimate the knowledge which young people possess and the responsibility which they exercise. As Rivers and Aggleton (1999) note, they may often behave more responsibly than their parents. While many young people begin sexual activity at a younger age than in earlier times, a large proportion abstain throughout adolescence or have a single partner, with females being typically less sexually active than males (Caraël, 1995).[5] Moreover, there is recent evidence in some cases of a reduction in risky behaviour. (UNAIDS 2000b).

When young women *are* sexually active, however, they often have older partners. In the era of AIDS, this heightens the danger they face, particularly if older men specifically seek them out in the belief that they are free from HIV infection. What is referred to as the 'sugar daddy' phenomenon involves sexual encounters not just across age but also income differentials, with young women suffering hardship, sometimes struggling to stay in school, agreeing to sexual relations in exchange for gifts, money or support (UNAIDS, 1998b), sometimes with the tacit acquiescence of their parents. The seriousness of the situation in some contexts is underlined by Fugle-sang's (1997) reference to girls as young as ten or eleven in Tanzania having sexual relations with men for chips, coke, money for videos or transport to school.

The danger posed to young women from sexual networking across generations also has repercussions for young men. The sentiment that they are a forgotten group in the equation, whose potential marital or sexual partners have been infected by an older group of men, was expressed in a rejoinder to a plea for renewed attention to the threat posed to millions of young African girls in or nearing their early teens: 'surely these young men also face an emergency? If they marry early and with a woman of their own age (or moderately younger), they are at considerable risk of being exposed to HIV' (af-aids:hivnet. 22.9.99). While 'young men also have a right to know the facts', it is evident that AIDS complicates patterns of conquest and of trust within and across lines of generation and gender.

Differences on the basis of marital status

Women's vulnerability to HIV is defined across lines not just of age but also of marital status. Young women may be at risk before marriage, but also within it, to the degree that their husbands wander (or, less commonly, that they themselves have sexual relations outside of marriage). Carpenter *et al.* (1997), for example, found that women aged 13–19 in Uganda who were HIV-positive were twice as likely to be married as those who were negative. The particular vulnerability of young married women follows from the way that desire for children makes protection problematic,[6] the fact that men tend to have more partners in the early years of marriage (Central Statistical Office [Zambia], 1997) and that husbands may be particularly prone to wander during their wife's pregnancy or in the first post-partum months (Leroy *et al.*, 1994; Cleland *et al.*, 1998).

Marriage is a context of considerable vulnerability for women in respect of HIV, because they can be infected, not through 'improper' behaviour, but in consequence of complying with norms of fidelity, if their husband has unprotected sex outside of marriage. However, if married women can be 'unwitting' recipients of HIV, their relative risk of infection is often less than that of women who are not married. Quigley *et al.* (1997), for example, found divorced and widowed women in rural communities in the Mwanza area of Tanzania three times more likely, than those currently married, to be HIV positive and, among those currently married, for the likelihood of infection to be higher among those previously divorced or widowed than those who had had a single marital partner.

These patterns may be partly a function of gender differences in the effects of HIV on marital partners. In general, it is men who bring HIV into a marriage, but in view of typical age differentials within marriage, women are infected at an earlier age. Given more rapid disease progression with age (UNAIDS, 1999g), husbands often die more quickly, leaving more widows (Rugalema, 1999). However, there is also a tendency for husbands who have lost their wives to remarry relatively quickly, in the process sometimes infecting their new partners. While the custom of widow inheritance persists in some places, potentially putting new husbands as well as remarried women in danger, increasingly widows are remaining unmarried. The situation of divorce is more complex, but here too there may sometimes be a direct connection with HIV. Data from a Ugandan study, for example, suggests that men are more likely than women to divorce partners who are HIV-positive and then to remarry (Carpenter *et al.*, 1999).

Divorced or widowed women often face severe economic hardship, which may be all the more stressful, should they themselves be ill or, in the case of widows, should they be subject to disinheritance or property grabbing.[7] With limited options they may turn to sex work, whether on an informal and casual basis or as a more formal means of securing livelihood. Or, they may resort to brewing beer or spirits, which attracts men who under the influence of alcohol are less than careful in sexual encounters. Whatever the case, they may generate suspicion and ill will on the part of married women, creating lines of division in blame and vindictiveness. Yet, while some women who are divorced or widowed – or single – have multiple partners and rely on commercial sex for their livelihoods, this is hardly true of all or even the majority of women in these categories (Gregson *et al.*, 1998).

Differences on the basis of income and access to services and resources

Early on in the AIDS epidemic in Africa, those who were better off and more highly educated seemed to be disproportionately affected. (Melbye *et al.*, 1986; Barnett and Blaikie, 1992). More recently Cohen (1998c) has characterised the epidemic as bi-modal in its effects, with peaks both among the richer and best educated and the poorest segments of the population. By virtue of their access to income and given their position in society, the 'non-poor', as he calls them, are afforded opportunities to engage in the sort of sexual behaviour which puts themselves, their families and their extra-marital partners at risk of HIV infection. This action of 'big men' (since this is more often true of men) is an expression of their power and largely a matter of choice. It contrasts with the situation of the poor – and especially poor women – whose poverty may lead them to exchange sexual favours for means of subsistence, but may also prevent or deter their taking preventive action.

Those who are better off and more highly educated – whether men and women – also have more access to information and to means of protection. There are limits to the ability to act on such information to ensure protection, particularly for women, given gendered power relations. However, evidence from Zambia suggests a levelling off in the incidence of new cases among those with higher levels of education, especially among young people (Fylkesnes *et al.*, 1997, 1999). It is hypothesised that those with more access to information are beginning to change their behaviour and to exercise choice in favour of protection (Fylkesnes *et al.*, 1999). Those who are better off also enjoy greater access to basic health care, better nutrition and, in some (albeit rare) cases, access to antiretroviral therapies.

In various ways, then, socio-economic position, gender, age and marital status intertwine to create a complex web of vulnerability. While there may be many points of mutual interest among those in different social locations, which affect change in behaviour, and many planes on which collective concerns can be articulated and mobilised, the dividing lines must also be acknowledged. Men and women face the epidemic from different standpoints. At the same time, however, women do not form a uniform category in respect of HIV/AIDS, nor do men. While experiencing a general vulnerability in consequence of gendered power relations, and the deep influence of ideologies of masculinity, the specific social location of specific women puts them in very different circumstances, sometimes in solidarity, but sometimes in opposition to one another. Men similarly may be generally subject to the harmful effects of an ideology of masculinity, which deters them from seeking knowledge and propels them into behaviours placing them at high risk of infection. However, at the same time they face one another through conflicting interests, as in the case of young men put at risk when their girlfriends and future wives are sought out and infected by older, more affluent men.

Interventions: towards prevention and increased protection

An understanding of the way the epidemic spreads and of the configuration of vulnerability it reveals and acts upon is essential to crafting effective means of protection. Yet interventions have not always been based on careful analysis of the dynamics of spread, nor have efforts always been as effective as hoped, or as required. There is an ongoing learning process in this regard, but many issues remain unresolved and under-researched. As Whelan (1999: 4) has commented, 'we know more about what needs to be done than we know how to do it'.

Our own focus on collective action at community level, and more specifically on women's contribution, is best seen within the context of competing discourses and a broader evolution of thinking about what makes interventions effective. This has involved a transition from reliance on medical knowledge and technologies, first towards an emphasis on behaviour, which alternatively facilitates or inhibits transmission and, second, towards consideration of the structural context in which behaviour occurs. We will briefly review this transition before giving more detailed consideration to collective action at community level on the part of women and the question of how far such interventions tackle the issue of gendered power relations.

From biomedicine to more integrated approaches

Medicine has experienced a series of triumphs, but also frustrations, with respect to AIDS. Early development of a test for the virus was crucial to documenting its presence and spread, with attendant possibilities for surveillance and control as well as identification of need. In practice, as Seidel (1993) notes, the infusion of a medical discourse into public policy tended to lend support towards control and coercion rather than towards rights and inclusiveness, and if this was more so in the early years, it has left a continuing legacy.

Contemporary medical preoccupations are more with treatment than with prevention, and more focused on the particular characteristics of the epidemic in the North than in the South. By virtue of market 'forces', important breakthroughs in antiretroviral therapies remain largely inaccessible to those other than the most privileged in poorer countries, particularly on the African continent. While energy is devoted to research on vaccines, and trials were in progress at the end of the century, there is less attention to those sub-types of HIV most common in the worst affected parts of Africa (Essex, 1999). Constrained by priorities of cost effectiveness and profitability and set within the context of limited medical infrastructure in many African settings, the focus of attention is rather on relatively inexpensive interventions, which could substantially reduce transmission of the virus from mothers to children (Gibb and Tess, 1999), a (selective) assault on STDs, whose presence greatly increases the probability of infection, and attempts to provide basic health care (UNAIDS, 1999e; World Bank, 1999). Given that so many in Africa remain without basic nutrition, access to HIV tests, adequate hospital facilities, drugs for the treatment of STDs or means to alleviate the symptoms of AIDS related conditions, the task even at this level, is enormous.

Medical science has retained hegemony at the level of discourse and in respect of budgetary decisions, and further medical breakthroughs continue to be hoped for. However, given the limits of medicine in halting the epidemic, particularly in Africa where cost factors and deficiencies of medical infrastructure restrict widespread utilisation of medicine's recent triumphs, the 'social side' of AIDS (Ankrah, 1991) has had to be addressed and prioritised. Initially, this involved an emphasis on public health. Subsequently the promotion of non-discrimination against those with HIV/AIDS was added, given recognition that stigma and high levels of surveillance did little to encourage prevention. Over time this in turn evolved into a broader concern with human rights. More recently there has been emphasis on the utility of integrating care and prevention. Taken together, these elements constitute what Whelan (1999) describes as a more strategic approach and what the document *Gender and HIV/AIDS* (UNAIDS, 1998b) refers to as an expanded response. It has implied an appreciation, not just of the need to attend to behaviour, but also the structural context in which behaviour occurs, including the gender ideologies and patterned relations which inform it.[8]

One way in which the notion of context or structure has entered into prescriptions for AIDS interventions is via the notion of enabling environments. Thus, in an overview of behavioural and social science in respect of AIDS, Des Jarlais and Caraël (1999: S236) warn against assuming that there will be 'heroic' behaviour change. Instead, they emphasise easing the way to risk reduction by attending to the context in which behaviour occurs. This may include changing policies, laws or increasing economic opportunities of those at high risk of infection and thereby most vulnerable. Campbell and Williams (1999) affirm the appropriateness of an enabling approach for the design of a project in Carletonville, South Africa, targeted at mineworkers and their partners, but involving the community as a whole. They define it as one which both seeks to remove structural barriers to health-protective action and attempts to fashion new structures which facilitate protective action or obstruct risk taking. In the case of the Carletonville project, they suggest, this might involve a focus on migrancy and housing, the economic dependence of women, high levels of rural poverty and existing safety legislation governing the mining industry.

Local initiatives: the case of women's groups

The Carletonville case illustrates not just an integrated approach which takes account of structural context, but a focus on community and local participation. Indeed a significant shift has occurred over the time of AIDS, from educational campaigns couched in individualistic terms toward community-based initiatives, paralleling a transition in development practice more generally from top-down, externally-led approaches towards those acknowledging the validity of local expertise (Bond and Vincent, 1997). This has entailed the designing of initiatives by or in collaboration with those most closely affected so as to modify or remove the constraints which they face (Rivers and Aggleton, 1999). A focus on women's groups and on harnessing women's organisational capacities in work around AIDS, whether in respect of care or prevention, is consistent with this broad advocacy of community-based initiatives. It follows from a concern to make full use of existing resources (Cohen and Reid, 1996) and acknowledges that women are not without power, influence or capabilities (Baylies and Bujra, 1995).

Ulin (1992: 67) has argued that 'women's collective perception of their ability to act on AIDS prevention messages could be a critical determinant of both male and female behaviour change'. Heise and Elias (1995: 940) concur, suggesting that women's history of rallying together to solve common problems represents an under-utilised strength in AIDS prevention campaigns. However, they develop further an argument alluded to by Ulin

(1992). Not only may women working together in a group be able to assist in AIDS work through increasing general awareness of the dangers of HIV, providing support for those living with HIV or AIDS or helping with the care of orphans. Their very involvement in such collective activity may also increase their awareness and give them strength to change their own behaviour or increase their capacity to negotiate for increased personal protection. In other words, such collective activity may both assist in meeting the group's formal objectives in respect of AIDS prevention and/or care and have an impact on members' consciousness and behaviour. It may be a vehicle for empowering its members in their own strategies of self preservation.

Heise and Elias (1995: 940) argue that by building group consensus within a community context, developing a unified sense of purpose, collectively reflecting on their situation and acting on their conclusions, a new sense of entitlement may emerge. They refer to the possibilities of spill-over into areas unrelated to an initial intervention. These points are illustrated with reference to a group of women whose prior experience in collective analysis gave them immediate confidence to discuss AIDS and to consider negotiating condom use with their partners, in stark contrast to a group lacking this prior experience, whose members were withdrawn and wary of even mentioning condoms to their husbands for fear of being beaten. But the principle may hold more generally that collective work around AIDS issues can have spill-over benefits for participants' own lives.

The key for Heise and Elias (1995) is not simply that individuals are organised in a group, but that the group learns and develops means of analysis, reflection and problem solving. The group becomes a vehicle for collective learning. This principle was validated by the work of Schoepf *et al.* (1991, 1993a) in Zaire. Based on the assumption that people already know a great deal about their own situation, 'experiential or process training', which Schoepf (1993a) had used elsewhere, was adapted to help in the development of a 'critical consciousness'. As she explains:

> We proposed to use action-research, an empowerment methodology, to enhance capacity of existing community groups and networks to undertake risk assessment and generate social support for behaviour change. We hypothesised that the method could be adapted readily to integrate HIV/AIDS prevention in programs of community development organisations' as well as other local groups.
>
> (Schoepf, 1993a: 1402)

Addressing gender relations

Such initiatives may be of considerable value in increasing levels of knowledge and awareness, improving negotiation skills, enhancing assertion and heightening self esteem. But how far can they also be effective in ensuring protection in the context of intimate relations? This remains an open – and critical – question. The problem is precisely the way gendered power relations, as configured in intimate relations, restrict the ability of women to secure their protection. The point has been made with considerable cogency (Hamlin and Reid, 1991; Heise and Elias, 1995; Sherr, 1996; Reid, 1997) that the trio of prevention strategies which have featured most predominantly in AIDS programmes – use of condoms, partner reduction and abstinence before marriage and fidelity within it – are inappropriate to the lives of many women. This is partly because they depend on co-operation with their male partners but also because, even if women may (and often do) control their own behaviour, they are unable to control that of their partners. It is this insight which has led to the critique of public health strategies which rely on individualistic models and, more particularly, which take insufficient notice of the broader context in which behaviour, and particularly gendered behaviour, occurs.

An examination of how and why the epidemic has gained so strong a grip has thus led to the deepest level of structures of inequality and injustice, along lines of gender, but also class and other social divisions. It has entailed a critique of prevailing structures and power relations at the level of the intimate social system, the society and the global political economy. For Hamlin and Reid (1991) this includes a critique of cultural practices, with identification of those which yield harmful consequences in the context of AIDS. To the extent that gender relations are implicated in this process, the very struggle against AIDS not only brings relations of gender inequality into question. It can also provide a persuasive basis for fundamental behavioural change. As de Bruyn (1992: 259) comments, strategies of protection against HIV have the ultimate capacity to serve as a 'platform' for furthering the emancipation of women in developing countries.

Reconciling short and long term objectives

Yet however compelling the analysis and however imperative the realisation that fundamental change is needed, in practice this cannot be immediately or comprehensively achieved. Hence, alongside recognition of the broader structural context, discussion of strategies of prevention and protection is often couched in terms of short term and long term initiatives and goals (Hamlin and Reid, 1991; de Bruyn, 1992; Ulin, 1992; Heise and Elias, 1995; Cohen and Reid, 1996; Rivers and Aggleton, 1998; UNAIDS, 1998b). As Rivers and Aggleton (1998) note, 'given the entrenched nature of existing gender roles, beliefs and expectations, it is unlikely that enormous advances can be made in the short term'. They therefore advocate an incremental approach 'which seeks to reduce the immediate risks of HIV infection within a gender sensitive framework'. Heise and Elias (1995: 931) advocate the need for far-reaching changes, including the establishing of new norms 'that stress mutuality, responsibility and equality between men and women' and a more equal sharing of power between men and women in both private and public spheres. However, they also acknowledge the need in the short term to protect women as far as possible while striving to enact such deeper changes, affirming the power and capacity which women exhibit and calling for more educational initiatives and attempts to effect changes in law and labour codes. Fundamental change takes time, they concede, but what must be done in the present is to begin the process of changing underlying causal factors and pursuing means to ensure protection *within* the context of current constraints.

This distinction between short and long term objectives has resonance with that made between practical and strategic gender interests in the broader development literature (Moser, 1993; Young, 1993; Kabeer, 1994; Karl, 1995). Drawn from analysis of political movements (Molyneux, 1985, 1998), these concepts underline dimensions of real and perceived power. Practical interests are those that follow from and are consistent with an existing gender division of labour and its associated structure of power. Policy or practice which is in accord with them (or indeed which advances them) eases current hardship, drudgery or the excesses of a prevailing pattern of gender relations without entailing fundamental change. Strategic interests, in contrast, are in accord with a vision of change, for example toward gender equality and justice unimpeded by gender divisions.

Planners have sometimes appropriated these concepts to accommodate predetermined agendas and externally formulated definitions of needs (Kabeer, 1994; Molyneux, 1998). Yet they remain useful for analysis of the nature and probable consequences of interventions and for assessing the extent to which a given initiative is consistent with perceived needs or interests and constitutes a viable 'fit' rather than an unrealistic intrusion. Most importantly, they are useful for examining how far short term interventions are consistent with and permit progress toward long term objectives. In the context of AIDS, long term, strategic, goals imply a transformation of prevailing gendered power relations and thereby an elimination of the inequalities making women especially vulnerable and putting women (and men) at risk. Interventions which meet practical, more immediate, interests of care and prevention can in some cases challenge existing structures and relations of power. However, they can alternatively consolidate them or have neutral impact. It is in order to separate out 'progressive' changes, that Young (1993) emphasises the importance of evaluating the transformative potential of interventions. Those which embody such potential need to be prioritised.

Using rather different language, but alluding to much the same principles, du Guerny and Sjöberg (1993) refer to 'gender traps' through which interventions around AIDS, which build on women's strength, may in some cases reinforce a prevailing gender division of labour. Over-reliance on women to provide care and support to those affected by HIV, for example, can thrust them back into traditional caring roles at the expense of achieving greater gender equality. By virtue of increasing women's burdens, such interventions can constrain women's capacity to push for the very structural changes which might secure their greater protection.

Emphasis on the need for coherence between short and long term objectives features strongly in the literature on gender and AIDS in developing countries. Thus, Hamlin and Reid (1991) caution that if strategies achievable in the short term do not address those inequalities which have given rise to the risk of infection, possibilities for more fundamental cultural and social change will be defused. Any potential conflict between long term and short term goals for women must thus be addressed, they argue, when formulating strategies around HIV/AIDS. However, lack of *full* engagement with such long term goals may also be at issue. It is on this basis, for example, that women-controlled methods of protection must be held up to critical appraisal.

Great store is sometimes put on the female condom or microbicides (Heise and Elias, 1995; Gottemoeller, 1999; Kaler, 1999) because they do not depend on men taking action and may offer some protection for women in predictably high risk situations. Yet these methods remain problematic on several levels. Although some research suggests increased acceptability (Madrigal *et al.*, 1998; Sinpisut *et al.*, 1998), the female condom is largely inaccessible, by virtue of price and availability, to the vast majority of women. As late as 1999, there had been no clinical studies assessing its effectiveness against HIV. Trials were still continuing on microbicides, with unresolved issues remaining as to their clinical efficacy and their safety (van Damme and Rosenberg, 1999). Were these difficulties to be overcome, questions would still remain as to how far these technologies permit control by women, and more specifically how far women could use them without their partner's knowledge and consent. A specific complaint about 'messiness' from both men and women in respect of microbicide trials (van Damme and Rosenberg, 1999) suggests that their covert use by women might well be problematic.

More importantly, such methods may side-step the underlying source of danger to women and the apparent control they permit may do little to shift the balance of power in intimate social systems, particularly if they are used covertly. As Heise and Elias (1995: 940) remark, they are 'no answer' and 'merely a ''band-aid'' for deeper problems in need of redress' insofar as they permit women to circumvent, but not alter, their lack of power in sexual relations (yet they also note that without such a band-aid, many may bleed to death before long term change can be effected.)

Linking spheres of empowerment: the importance of economic security

One of our primary concerns is how far women's groups involved in AIDS work can become vehicles not just for collective learning but for 'empowerment' and, if so, how and in what ways this becomes manifest in participants' lives. An important corollary is how far they achieve the expanded vision referred to in *Gender and HIV/AIDS* (UNAIDS, 1998b) linking protective strategies with broader goals, i.e. a linking of short with long term objectives. Interventions aimed at increasing levels of AIDS awareness and improving negotiation skills through the vehicle of women's groups may have theoretical consistency with long term goals of modifying or transforming gender relations. However, are there other aspects of women's collective work around AIDS which can progress this further? How far does the link between women's position within intimate social systems and the wider society need also to be explicitly addressed?

One aspect of this involves women's economic dependence which figures so strongly as a factor of vulnerability, reinforced by the broad fabric of gender relations at both a societal level and within the confines of relations of intimacy. Specifically, how does women's involvement with community initiatives around AIDS intersect with their economic situation? Might any 'empowerment' or improved negotiation skills gained through group experience or collective learning be negated (and its enactment or practice inhibited) by continuing economic dependence on partners? Do women even have sufficient economic security to spare time for AIDS related activities, given the economic constraints many face?

The contradictions described by these questions have frequently prompted the combining of AIDS work with income generating activities by women's groups. Links have been drawn between women's increasing economic independence and their decision making power within households, which, it is sometimes claimed, may correlate positively with greater control over fertility and, by extension, have positive implications for a general shift in the balance of decision making in intimate relations to ensure greater protection against AIDS (UNAIDS, 1998b). However, all of this is tenuous, indeed almost speculative, and supportive evidence is sparse. Whelan's (1999: 26) review reveals the paucity of studies which attempt to measure the impact of particular interventions. Even those few which he cites tend to be concerned more with women's broad social and economic status than specifically linked to AIDS. While he subsequently notes that 'a number of community-based organisations are implementing programmes that incorporate both economic development and HIV/AIDS focused activities (Whelan, 1999: 29), he also remarks that few have been evaluated. This remains a challenge for the future.

Limits of women-only approaches?

Given the enormity of the task, enthusiasm for the potential of women's collective action to make an important contribution to work around AIDS is frequently qualified by the insistence that women-only action is insufficient or that women can not stop the AIDS epidemic on their own. Thus, Ulin (1992: 64), so forceful in support of harnessing women's organisational capabilities, completes her assertion that 'the solidarity of women in rural African communities may be their greatest source of strength for coping with the AIDS epidemic' with the rejoinder, 'but they cannot cope alone. They must be empowered to share the responsibility with men, participating equally in personal and community strategies to block transmission of the virus'. Subsequently, she reinforces the point: 'nevertheless, women's empowerment is only half the solution: men too must acknowledge their joint responsibility, and all members of the society must be willing to redefine sexual roles in relation to the health of the family and the community' (Ulin, 1992: 67). Cohen and Reid (1996) similarly insist that 'there can be no individual solutions' and that 'men have to be active agents as well as women'.

While there may be broad agreement that men and women must work together, that men must be brought on board, that co-operation is necessary – and that all of this is logically consistent with the fundamental structural change required to stem the epidemic – the way in which this is to be achieved often remains vague and unspecified. Thus, admonitions are offered blandly, almost as truisms. The document *Women and AIDS, Agenda for Action*, issued under the auspices of the WHO (1995) just prior to the Beijing inter-national conference on women, argues for example that 'if the vulnerability of women to HIV infection is to be reduced, both men and women must work to counter gender discrimination and the subordination of women'. However, it provides little elaboration of mechanisms to effect this. Declaring that 'UNAIDS speaks out for safer, egalitarian norms', the document *Women and AIDS* (UNAIDS, 1997) suggests empowerment as an antidote and lists 'six paths to empowerment' as comprising combating ignorance, providing women-friendly services, developing female controlled prevention methods, reinforcing women's economic independence, and reducing vulnerability through political change. But issues of sequencing, the interconnection between these various elements and the most effective entry points remain to be theorised and specified.

Male responsibility

An increasingly common corollary to the thesis that women on their own cannot effect the change needed to halt the advance of AIDS is that greater attention should be directed toward men. Indeed, a central plank of Foreman's (1999) argument is that the AIDS epidemic is driven by men, given that the 'core group' in respect of AIDS, defined as those both liable to contract and transmit the virus, is comprised of men. It is not this central fact, however, so much as self interest, which Foreman and others frequently call on as a mechanism for inducing change. If women are at risk from current sexual norms, undergirded by ideologies of masculinity, so too are men (Ankrah, 1991; Rivers and Aggleton, 1998; UNAIDS, 1998b, Foreman, 1999). Thus, there have been suggestions that aspects of ideologies of masculinity need to be both engaged with and modified in ways which are more productive of safety. de Bruyn (1992), for example, has recommended the delinking of condoms from family planning and their use being emphasised as 'manly';

and indeed marketing has reflected insight on the way in which prevailing discourses can be both utilised and manipulated to induce product acceptance (and, by the by, increased profitability). There may also be possibilities for rethinking notions of maleness so that strength becomes associated with maturity and self control, questioning the view that men's sexuality is beyond their control or that conquest is a necessary and valued attribute of manliness (Bujra, 2000c).

In practice, the most common approach, has been to emphasise male responsibility, as indicated in the subtitle of the book *AIDS and men, taking risks or taking responsibility* (Foreman, 1999). As Fuglesang (1997) notes, the theme of responsibility figured prominently in the 1994 Cairo conference on population and development, which emphasised both women's rights and the necessity of men being brought into fertility decisions and family planning, through accepting a responsible role and in turn being treated as responsible partners. This theme is strongly pursued by Cohen and Reid (1996), who indeed place responsibility on a plane higher than rights, at least with respect to men's basket of rights and responsibilities. Men, they suggest, need to recognise the consequences of their acts and behave responsibly both in their own interests and those of their family. This sense that men's role as responsible partners and parents can be invoked in AIDS campaigns has been taken up by Rivers and Aggleton (1998) who comment that 'the concern which many men express about the health and welfare of their children may provide a useful way of gaining attention in relation to HIV-related work'.

Gender sensitive but woman-centred?

While offering a 'way in' to reflection about what it means to be a partner, husband or father (or son), the varied components of male roles and the meaning of 'maleness', such approaches, whether appealing to self interest or to paternalistic responsibilities, may be of limited *transformative* value insofar as they maintain and indeed consolidate male control, initiative and dominance. There has been a tendency in the recent past to co-opt a women's agenda, sometimes in the name of gender, whether in respect of development writ large or more specific health or population goals, which must surely be resisted in strategies designed to counter the AIDS epidemic. Elson (1995) has noted that arguments for removing male bias may be couched either as pragmatism or as principles of equity and justice. In the short run, it is in the interests of governments within developing countries to remove barriers to women's economic participation which inhibit full utilisation of productive forces. However, this may have little to do with the emancipation of women. A much remarked upon correlation between women's literacy and rates of fertility (Kabeer, 1994; Sadik 1994) has directed attention at improving women's education, not so much for the sake of women, but in order to better achieve goals of population policy. Beneath such slogans as 'educate a woman and you educate the nation' is a displacement of a woman's fulfilment or realisation of her capabilities in favour of the interests of her children and the development of a nation's 'human resources'.

Some of the initiatives in the field of AIDS prevention and care have had this flavour as well, taking note of women's capabilities and then placing greater burdens on them, rather than focusing on women as people in their own right, with specific needs. A move towards men's involvement and partnership is in part a pragmatic realisation that there are precisely limits, given gendered power relations, to what women can achieve. However, it is crucial that support for this shift does not lose sight of the need for mutuality. In identifying men's self interest, it is important that strategies of protection against HIV do not simply reinforce men's paternalistic role as responsible for – rather than as *equally* responsible *with* – women.

Conclusions

While self interest needs to be highlighted, it is crucial that the mutuality of interests of men and women be kept at the forefront of any strategy. It is gender *relations*, the position, interaction, rights and responsibilities of *both* women and men, which are pivotal. It is important to resist those apparently gender sensitive approaches which simply shift their focus from women to men – or from a female to a male perspective – and to insist on maintaining a woman-centred approach in AIDS work (Reid, 1997). While partnership, co-operation, mutual reflection and problem solving which cross boundaries of gender – as well as age and other lines of social division – are necessary, the relative disadvantage of women requires that they retain the initiative as far as possible in any programme, project or intervention. Any intervention, more-over, must be fashioned with full appreciation for how it impacts on existing patterns of gender relations and there must be care to ensure that it serves to *progress* the process of ensuring greater equality and justice. It is crucial that it be not merely consistent with the sort of transformations deemed necessary for ensuring protection, but nudges the process along.

In what follows we explore a range of questions thrown up by this analysis. Women's vulnerability may apply in general by virtue of gender relations manifest in both public and private spheres. However, what needs to be demonstrated is how they configure in particular situations, in view of specific economic constraints and (changing) cultural prescriptions. Women's collec-tive responses have emerged in many settings in relation to the crisis posed by AIDS. How have they fared? How far have they succeeded in mobilising women's strengths? To what extent do divisions among women – on the basis of generation, religion, ethnicity or class – impede their impact? How far have women's groups contributed to campaigns of protection or the provision of care? How far have they impacted directly on the lives of their members? To what extent have the activities of such groups addressed the underlying gender relations which fuel the epidemic? To what extent and how successfully have men been brought into collective initiatives? How far have initiatives reconciled short term objectives with an ultimate need to transform the way in which gender relations create vulnerability to HIV infection for both women and men? It is such issues which guide our analysis of the experience of communities and AIDS organisations in Tanzania and Zambia.

Notes

1   Note must be taken of problems of comparability of data across countries in respect of the continuity and scope of surveillance testing upon which estimates are based. In most cases in Africa, for example, the date for the most recent prevalence data for women attending antenatal care clinics in major urban centres is prior to 1997 for 16 countries and missing altogether for two others. (UNAIDS, 2000c).

2   For example, de Bruyn (1992) comments that in Botswana AIDS is sometimes referred to as a pollution disease originating in the female body and transferred to men during culturally proscribed periods, including after birth, abortion, or before ritual cleansing.

3   See also Ankrah *et al.* (1996) and Macwan'gi *et al.* (1994) on women as carers in the context of AIDS.

4   There may be questions about the universality of such capabilities as well as the appropriateness of means of their measurement, either via the gender related development index or any other tool. Authors of the Human Development Report (1995: 102) acknowledge that preferences and the interpretation of some rights may differ, depending on cultural traditions and assert that 'there should be no attempt to offer a universal model of gender equality', even while offering their index as a means of estimating the lapses of such equality.

5   According to data reviewed by Caraël (1995) for nine African countries, between 46 and 90 per cent of males and between 44 and 97 per cent of females aged 15–19 reported having had no sexual intercourse during the previous 12 months. Of those who did, the average number of partners (for six of the nine countries for which data was available) ranged from 1.0 to 1.9 for females and from 1.6 to 2.5 for males. The average number of sexual partners during the previous 12 months for the age group taken as a whole ranged from 0.0 to 0.5 for females and 0.2 to 0.9 for males.

6   Although during this same period, when not actually trying for a child, they may be more able to negotiate the use of a condom for the purposes of family planning.

7   The term refers to a custom whereby property of a husband is claimed by his relatives on his death, often leaving widows and surviving children in great difficulty. While often illegal in respect of civil marriage (e.g. in the case of Zambia), and publicly condemned, instances of the practice continue.

8   See also Tawil *et al.* (1999) who define an expanded vision of HIV prevention as incorporating both risk reduction strategies and social, economic and policy interventions.

2 Responses to the AIDS epidemic in Tanzania and Zambia

Janet Bujra and Carolyn Baylies

The specific nature of the AIDS epidemic varies from place to place, depending on historical circumstance, cultural context and contemporary political economy. Moreover, within any given locality it may appear as a series of superimposed epidemics (Lindenbaum, 1992), marking out fractures along lines of gender, generation or other social divisions. As Kreniske (1997) has observed, disease is a social event, which expresses the central realities of the society in which it occurs. Given its social embeddedness, this applies with particular transparency in the case of AIDS. As well as highlighting internal flaws and weak points in the social fabric (Santana, 1997), however, AIDS also exposes relations of dependence between countries, particularly where poverty makes some susceptible to the ostensibly benevolent, but also potentially intrusive, influence of donors and international non-governmental organisations (NGOs) As Lindenbaum (1992: 330) suggests, a full rendering of the epidemic requires that it be placed not just in local context, but within the 'geopolitics of competing international communities'.

While acknowledging these layers of influence and meaning, this chapter focuses on the national level – given that it is here that policy is formulated – in providing a background for the six studies of community and organisational experience covered in subsequent chapters. While the history of AIDS is specific to each country – and within it to each community – there are many points of commonality for the two countries dealt with here, shared in turn with other countries in the region. The fact that the AIDS epidemic is framed by the politics of development and by the dependent and wretched place of many African nations within the global political economy accounts for many similarities in policy and practice. Both Tanzania and Zambia have experienced severe economic crises, imposed structural adjustment packages requiring privatisation and the introduction of user fees for social services and externally dictated planning frames with sometimes contradictory emphases on co-ordination, decentralisation and multisectorality.

Tanzania's population is three and a half times that of Zambia's, but the two countries have similar demographic structures with about 45 per cent in the age range 15–45. Although there are diverse local languages spoken within both countries, Swahili, as Tanzania's official language, is understood by virtually all within its boundaries, while English, as the official language of Zambia, is only understood by some of its citizens, often a minority in the rural areas. Both countries rank low on UNDP's 2000 Human Development and Gender-related Development Indices, with Zambia's position at 153 and Tanzania's 156 on each among a total of 174 countries (UNDP, 2000). Tanzania has a lower *per capita* income, but this may exaggerate the difference in standard of living between the two. A higher proportion of Zambia's population is urbanised, at 44 per cent in 1997 as against just 26 per cent in Tanzania (World Bank, 1998) and declines in rural self sufficiency in Zambia may even out some of the apparent differences in income between the two.[1] On the other hand, a higher rate of urbanisation in Tanzania points to levels of mobility, which can constitute a particular hazard in the era of AIDS.[2] Zambia has a higher adult literacy rate than Tanzania and a greater proportion of its young population enrolled in schools, but a lower average life expectancy (UNDP, 2000), which under the impact of AIDS is likely to dip further.

In the early years of independence, Tanzania's government emphasised the importance of self-reliance and collective development effort, principles which were subsequently taken up, although to perhaps a lesser extent, in Zambia. The histories of both countries include episodes of strong resistance to external pressures, support for liberation movements in the region and antagonism to the structural adjustment policies of international institutions. Yet both have succumbed (with varying degrees of grace) to external regimes of financial control and both are highly indebted. By 1996 total external debt stood at 114 per cent of Tanzania's annual gross national product, while the figure for Zambia was 161 per cent (World Bank, 1998).

These features provide the backdrop to the impact of AIDS. The populations of both countries faced problems of day to day survival and extensive obstacles to development without this added complication. The spread of AIDS within them has been exacerbated by low levels of nutrition, poor health infrastructure and general difficulties of getting by. In turn, the epidemic constitutes a significant threat to future development prospects (Baylies, 1999b).

In what follows, the story of the epidemic's spread throughout each country is first recounted. Responses to the epidemic by governments and civil society are then reviewed, with consideration given to both strengths and limitations. In examining policy and practice, a key concern is the extent to which gender figures in local discourses around AIDS and in policies oriented towards prevention. In an appendix to the chapter we describe the methodology employed in our investigation of gender and AIDS and introduce the specific sites where the research was conducted, identifying the themes taken up in the account of each.

First diagnoses and unfolding patterns of prevalence

The beginnings of the AIDS epidemic in Zambia and Tanzania, as elsewhere, are difficult to pinpoint. As a Zambian doctor noted, the fact that HIV was identified in the industrialised world and initially associated with homosexuality and injecting drug use clouded the picture, so that it was 'unthinkable' for any doctor in the early 1980s to say unequivocally that it was present locally (Mukonde, 1992). AIDS was first officially diagnosed in Zambia in 1984 and declared a major public health threat in 1986,[3] but Mukonde notes that several patients in the early 1980s had symptoms compatible with what would later be clinically diagnosed as AIDS.[4] In Tanzania, the first cases of AIDS were diagnosed in 1983 in the Bukoba district, where the country borders on Uganda.

Once formally acknowledged, recorded cases of HIV and AIDS increased rapidly in both countries, although always underreported, given the lack of diagnostic facilities, the shame and fear preventing many from seeking a diagnosis and the prohibitive cost to some of seeking care. The progress of the epidemic, however, was quickly reflected in the strain it inflicted on the health services. In 1986, 13 per cent of consecutive admissions to some of Zambia's urban hospitals were AIDS-related, with the proportion increasing as early as 1989 to 35 per cent (Mudenda, 1991). Early tests were not always reliable, confounding the task of estimating prevalence. In Tanzania, the cumulative number of reported AIDS cases rose to 25,503 in 1990, to 81,498 in 1995 and to 109,863 in 1998 (NACP, 1999). In Zambia the total number of reported cases of AIDS and AIDS Related Complex was 44,942 by 1997 (Ministry of Health, NASTLP, 1997). The actual numbers are much higher. UNAIDS' estimates of cumulative totals of AIDS cases, derived from models and based largely on surveillance testing of attendants of antenatal clinics, were 1,000,000 for Tanzania and 770,000 for Zambia at the end of 1997 (UNAIDS, annexes, 1998c) while the estimated number of those living with HIV or AIDS was at the end of 1999, 1,300,000 and 870,000, respectively (UNAIDS, 2000c).[5]

In both countries, the mode of HIV transmission is predominantly heterosexual (over 92 per cent), although there are also many cases of transmission from mother to child. AIDS is a serious health and development problem in each, indeed a developmental emergency, but its impact may be greater in Zambia where the estimated rate of prevalence among adults is about twice as high (at about 19.95 per cent at the end of 1999) as in Tanzania (8.09 per cent). There is accordingly a higher estimated proportion of orphans in Zambia than Tanzania, but given differences in total population, this translates into a larger number in Tanzania (at a cumulative total of 1,100,000 by the end of 1999) than Zambia (650,000) (UNAIDS/WHO, 2000a,b).

Within and between Zambia and Tanzania, AIDS has moved along transport arteries, both major and minor (see Box 1). In Tanzania it seems to have moved from Kagera towards Dar es Salaam and then outwards to other regions. While initial diagnoses in Zambia were made in the capital's teaching hospital, patients were sometimes referred there from provincial centres (Mukonde, 1992). Given the incubation period of the virus and the delay in recognition of the syndrome, precise paths of the epidemic are difficult to reconstruct. Spreading through sexual networks involving spouses, friends and 'strangers', prevalence has been higher the more members of a given population are on the move. Lorry drivers on transnational routes and long distance traders have been implicated in both countries as transmitters of the virus. Such travellers may have a series of regular or casual partners along their routes, with commercial sex burgeoning to meet expanding demand. Transit stops have thus become HIV 'hotspots'. In both Zambia and Tanzania, many of these are near international borders – such as Livingstone and Chipata in Zambia or Mwanza and Mbeya in Tanzania – where prevalence may be higher than in some larger urban areas within each country. But there are others, such as Serenje and Kapiri Mposhi within Zambia, where drivers en route to East Africa, South Africa, Malawi or Zaire pause in their travels (Chalowandya and Chitomfwa, 1995a). Particular commercial circuits, such as the fish trade between the northern part of Luapula Province and Zambia's Copperbelt (Mushingeh *et al.*, 1990–1991) or trade in vegetables in the vicinity of Lushoto, may also constitute routes for the passage of HIV, particularly when the exchange of sex becomes crucial to entry into business.

Box 2.1 Liaisons on the train from Tanzania to Zambia – passages of HIV

The following account comes from the research diary of Julius Mwabuki (June, 1995). It recounts a disagreement among *young people* in Lushoto town about who was most responsible for the spread of AIDS.

Juliana questioned Eric's view, that women were killing men with AIDS. Her opinion was that it was men, or that both were killing each other. Men demanded sex from women without gaining their consent. Eric's response was: 'Why do you agree if you are not stupid? You have the right to say no'. 'It depends,' replied Juliana, 'sometimes men force women'. In an endeavour to convince his companions, Eric related the following account of an experience he had on a train from Tanzania to the seminary in Zambia where he was training for the priesthood.

Having taken his seat in a first class cabin, he was surprised to discover that his companion was a young lady. This was a sleeper for two people and normally unmarried people of opposite sex were never placed together. The basis of the error became clear when he glanced at his ticket and realised that his first name was written there as Erica. However, he was reluctant to report the matter because the lady was very beautiful. As he and his companion sat staring at one another, there was a knock on the door and a policewoman entered. She was shocked to discover the two of them within the cabin, but in response to her predictable question, Eric, having gained confidence, told her that the young woman was his wife. The policewoman requested to see their certificate of marriage, whereupon Eric changed his story and said she was actually his girlfriend, whom he expected to marry. He signalled to the young woman, who was looking decidedly perplexed, to keep silent. Apparently satisfied, the policewoman left. The young lady now revealed herself to be very displeased, but Eric pleaded with her to cool down, or else she might be transferred to third class. Shortly thereafter a policeman came by the cabin and he, too, expressed mild astonishment at their presence together in the cabin. Eric now became more assertive: 'You guys, what is the matter? Is it funny to travel with my wife-to-be?' The policeman was not inclined to argue the point and merely asked to see their tickets. He satisfied himself that they were both in the right cabin and noted that the name on his passenger list was indeed Eric. However, he was puzzled by the fact that Eric's destination was listed as Zambia and the young woman's as Tunduma, Tanzania. Quick on his feet, Eric explained that she was stopping to visit her parents for a few days before joining him in Zambia. The policeman accepted this story and went on his way.

Once alone, the young woman informed Eric that she had a husband in Dar es Salaam. 'Why are you defending yourself,' Eric asked. 'What is the matter?' She replied that she was afraid of being disturbed: 'you guys are so stupid'. Somewhat taken aback, Eric decided to go out for some beer. He returned with three bottles and offered her one but was shocked when she said that she drank more than one beer at a time. When she realised that a second bottle was not forthcoming, she left, saying she was going to the buffet. She was gone for some time and Eric eventually fell asleep. He was woken when she returned and demanded that he tell the drunken man who was with her that Eric was her husband. The man was disturbing her, she said, simply because she had accepted two beers from him.

Eric was startled by the turn of events but accepted that since he had created the falsehood he had to defend it. He tried his level best to chase the man away but the drunken man insisted that he be repaid for the beers with sex. At a loss, Eric went in search of the police. Fortunately, the policewoman was not very far away, and he told her about the problem. Returning, they found the cabin locked, but they could hear screams from inside. When they were able to open the door using a spare key, it was clear that the man was trying to rape the young woman, and he was summarily arrested.

Back in the cabin after all the trouble, the young woman told him the truth – that she was a student going home for holidays. Gradually the atmosphere warmed. However, Eric was now very tired and wanted to sleep. The young woman was unhappy about this and complained of feeling cold. Eric tried to ignore her, but then she came across to join him on his side of the cabin. This placed Eric in a state of some agitation. He was worried even to touch her, but was caught 'helpless' when she turned on his radio cassette and requested a dance. He was 'forced' to dance with her, but as he did so his sense of unease increased. He had no condom with him and he worried that he would not be able to prevent himself from unsafe sex. Nor in the event was he.

At the end of his story his companions mulled over what he had said. One asked whether this was truly the end and whether they still see one another. Eric said they have met since, but did not trust one another.

HIV has also been transported to rural areas by migrants to the cities or to centres of commerce who have returned when ill. Indeed one of the vernacular names for AIDS in Zambia translates as 'go home and say good bye to your mother'.[6] In the hamlets around Lushoto and in the Kilimanjaro region of Tanzania (Bujra, 2000c; Setel, 1996), AIDS is seen as an affliction brought back by returning migrants, with resentment expressed either against the 'big' business people who move back and forth between the area or younger members of the community who 'run off' to towns and come back ill. But in most provincial centres and many rural areas, AIDS is increasingly seen as 'among us' rather than a curse inflicted by strangers or prodigal sons and daughters.

Given the unevenness of reporting year on year,[7] descriptions of prevalence patterns within each country must be advanced with caution, as must any comparisons drawn between them. However, rates in Zambia's major urban centres have been generally higher than those in Tanzania. In 1997, extrapolated estimates of adult prevalence were above 25 per cent in the urban sectors of most districts across Zambia and 30 per cent or higher in Lusaka, as well as in Eastern Province. At the same time Zambia has been characterised by a clear urban-rural differential in respect of AIDS. In 1997, for example, overall urban adult prevalence was estimated at 27.9 per cent and rural prevalence at 14.8 per cent. (Ministry of Health, Zambia, 1997). In Tanzania the picture is more complicated. While it is clear that prevalence is low in many rural areas and even urban centres within some regions, it is very high in both the urban centres and rural sections of particular districts. A case in point is Kagera and especially the Bukoba district, where AIDS was first reported, although it now appears to be levelling off (Tibaijuka, 1997; Msamanga, 1999).[8] It is also concentrated in Mbeya Urban and some districts of Mbeya Rural, and in Iringa and Rukwa (NACP, 1996).

In both countries AIDS has cut a swathe through the youngest and the fittest. Its effects are concentrated in the age group 20–44, the period of prime economic, social and sexual adult activity. As the Annual Report of Tanzania's National AIDS Control Programme notes, 'AIDS is killing many of the productive force of the population' (NACP, 1998b: 13; Tibaijuka, 1997). In Tanzania, the largest number of AIDS cases among men are in the age range 30–39 and among women 20–29. (UNAIDS, 1998d). In Zambia the pattern is broadly similar.

While prevalence may be lower, females under the age of 25 are particularly vulnerable and incidence in this age group particularly high. Surveys of attendants at ante-natal clinics in Zambia in 1994, for example, revealed prevalence rates of more than 20 per cent among women aged 15–19 at some urban sites (NASTLP, n.d.),[9] and it has been reported that the greater number of all new infections were within this age category (Fylkesnes, 1995). This accords with a prospective study in Dar es Salaam, Tanzania showing highest incidence in this group among women attending family planning clinics (Kapiga *et al.*, 1998).

Early responses to AIDS: fascination, fear and denial

People in Tanzania and Zambia first heard about AIDS as a deadly disease which was happening somewhere else, among other people. When its presence was confirmed locally, it was greeted with the same sense of panic and attempts to apportion blame as occurred in other settings. One of the earliest reports in the Zambian press, in 1985, was of a 28 year old Zambian woman living in Australia who, 7 months pregnant, was admitted to hospital and found to be suffering from AIDS. The reports followed her return to Zambia to give birth at the University Teaching Hospital, where there was tight security borne of worries about the spread of infection. Upon her discharge the permanent secretary of the Ministry of Health found it necessary to reassure the population, telling them not to panic. A nurse who had refused to attend the woman in hospital was suspended from her duties (*Times of Zambia*, 24 May 1985; 6 July 1985; 9 July 1985; 10 July 1985; and 12 July 1985). A sense of deep anxiety and uncertainty infused much early reporting, with headlines of stories in the Zambian press in 1985 declaring 'AIDS worries Zambian health personnel', 'disease is a puzzle', 'bedbugs AIDS carriers' and 'can I get AIDS from a mosquito?' In Tanzania a reader's letter to the *Sunday News* in 1986 (7 April) worried that imported second-hand clothing could spread HIV.

The setting up and evolution of national AIDS programmes

Politicians and government officials were initially reluctant to admit the presence of AIDS, but towards the end of 1985, the Zambian government made a formal announcement to this effect. The following year a National AIDS Surveillance Committee and an inter-sectoral AIDS Health Education

Committee were established and charged with co-ordinating the control and prevention of HIV/AIDS within the country. With the assistance of WHO, a National AIDS/STD/Tuberculosis and Leprosy Programme (NASTLP)[10] was set up and in July 1987, an emergency short term plan was launched. Its primary aim was to ensure a safe supply of blood within the country, but it also provided guidelines for clinical diagnosis and management of AIDS patients and initiated an AIDS awareness campaign. A 5 year medium term plan was subsequently put into place, covering the period 1988 through 1993 (NASTLP, 1994).

A similar pattern of events unfolded in Tanzania, reflecting a relatively rapid response to the threat posed by AIDS. Within 2 years of the first confirmed cases, an initial Task Force was set up which was formalised as the National AIDS Control Programme (NACP) in 1988. Its prime objective was to monitor the progress of the epidemic, drawing on regular testing of blood donors and women attending ante-natal clinics, and to issue annual reports. As in Zambia, the NACP was also charged with organising the distribution of disposable needles and condoms. Another of its key tasks was to initiate public health campaigns in an attempt to slow down the spread of AIDS, focusing particularly on youth and on family life education. To facilitate this work it was directed to stimulate research and to disseminate research findings (NACP, 1998b).

In both countries, national programmes have been subject to a series of reviews and in some respects found wanting, necessitating rethinking and re-orientation. The World Bank's (1992) *AIDS Assessment and Planning Study* in Tanzania was critical of the limited development of the AIDS programme there, arguing that its efforts were spread too thinly, and that it had not been given effective top level support. Similar points emerged from a consensus workshop held in Zambia in May 1993 involving representatives of NGOs, government and the donor community held prior to the launching of the country's second medium term AIDS plan. It recommended more education and behavioural change at the individual level. However, it also drew attention to those structural and cultural factors facilitating transmission, which impinged on but were outside the immediate control of individuals (NASTLP, 1994).

In Zambia this signalled a shift, in line with a broader transition in thinking about AIDS at the international level, from concern with risk behaviour to a focus on vulnerability as situated in relations of power and access to resources. Concern for women was particularly highlighted and their vulnerability to HIV explained in structural terms: low levels of literacy impeding access to information, economic dependence on men and susceptibility to infection in consequence of certain cultural practices. A document produced at the time elaborated upon these issues, with reference to both social and biological factors affecting women's vulnerability to HIV (Ministry of Health, Zambia, 1993). It argued for an approach going beyond medical interventions to incorporate legal change, education and economic empowerment. Also affirmed at this juncture was the need for community-based interventions to employ participatory approaches (NASTLP, 1994). In Tanzania, though there were similar references to community action and cultural factors, the importance of an understanding of gender relations went officially unacknowledged, even as late as 1998 (NACP, 1998c).

The national AIDS programmes in both countries have realised significant achievements. In Tanzania, a policy document was produced in 1996 which underlined the right to confidentiality of AIDS sufferers and the illegality of pre-employment HIV testing or of discrimination at work against people with AIDS (*Daily News*, 6 May 1996). The NACP also proposed that politicians, lawyers and government officials be made aware of the political, social and legal issues relating to AIDS. A network of lawyers, doctors and policy makers was set up to look at the ethical issues raised by AIDS and to monitor human rights abuses (*AIDS Analysis Africa*, 7 February 1997).

A mid-term review of Zambia's second medium term plan, conducted in early 1997 (Republic of Zambia, 1997) commended the way in which the NASTLP had commissioned research in key areas, compiling a useful store of data and generating considerable insight. It acknowledged that there had been greatly increased awareness of AIDS issues among the general population and greater readiness to speak about sexual behaviour. However, it also pointed to many constraints and difficulties, including understaffing of the national AIDS office, a general lack of national policies on AIDS, patchy enforcement of existing legislation, and limited enactment of a multi-sectoral approach. Similar conclusions were reached in a review of the Tanzanian situation prior to the enactment of the third medium term plan on HIV/AIDS. Although formal lipservice has been paid to multisectorality, in practice the fight against AIDS has continued to be seen primarily as a health issue (NACP, 1998a: 7; Msamanga, 1999).

Responses from civil society with support from external sources

Nudging government along, complementing and sometimes substituting for official programmes, have been efforts by mission hospitals, churches, NGOs, community-based organisations and concerned individuals. This response has reflected a genuine outpouring of compassion and concern for fellow human beings as well as an attempt to channel anxiety in productive ways and gain some control over an unwelcome and frightening threat to well-being. The dynamics of these non-official or non-governmental responses bear some resemblance to those which occurred in North America and Europe during this same period. In the African context, however, community action was not so much a consequence of the vacuum left by governments, initially unwilling to acknowledge the threat of the crisis and to come to the aid of a section of the population already stigmatised by what some regarded as aberrant sexuality. There *was* considerable denial among the ranks of government officers in African countries, as elsewhere, followed by scapegoating and finger pointing. However, the fundamental problem was less unwillingness to act than lack of resources, exacerbated even further by the effects of structural adjustment directives.

Collective action at community level has been encouraged in Tanzania and Zambia, as across much of the continent, precisely *because* of the limited capacity of governments to meet the needs engendered by the emergency.[11] However, those at the 'grassroots' are also hampered by limited resources. Some initiatives have therefore drawn on existing organisations, informal networks or NGOs. Some have obtained assistance from the donor community. Several examples can serve to illustrate how early in the epidemic a range of specific interventions were devised and put in place.

Early initiatives

One of the first large-scale initiatives around AIDS in Zambia was the Anti-AIDS Project, which encouraged the formation of anti-AIDS clubs in schools and tertiary institutions. It began in 1986[12] as a follow-on from a talk by an expatriate doctor to students at a Lusaka secondary school, prompted by their teachers' concern.[13] With sponsorship from the Norwegian aid agency (NORAD), a small team began to organise competitions on AIDS prevention themes and produce materials which were distributed freely to anyone wishing to make use of them. The idea of forming clubs to discuss and disseminate information about AIDS caught on and numbers quickly mushroomed, with 1767 being registered by 1994.[14]

Another early initiative was the Copperbelt Health Education Project (CHEP), which remains the most important AIDS NGO on the Zambian Copperbelt. One of its founders was a young Indian doctor, V. Chandra Mouli, who had come to Zambia to practice medicine in 1982. As the threat of AIDS became ever more immediate, he argued for a concerted education effort. CHEP was initially linked to the Kitwe Branch of Rotary International, drawing thereby on the charitable concerns of better-off members of the local community. In November 1988 it became an independent NGO, largely funded by NORAD and supported by the NASTLP. From the beginning it worked in alliance with other local groups and made use of existing resources, such as materials produced by the Anti-AIDS Project, adapting them as appropriate (Mouli, 1991, 1992).

As well as prevention, efforts were extended to care and counselling. One of the first examples of what became a continent-wide initiative was the home-based care programme developed at the Salvation Army's Chikankata Hospital in Zambia's Southern Province (Campbell, 1989; Chela *et al.*, 1989; Campbell and Williams, 1990; Williams 1990). It was devised in 1987 as an outreach service, involving a team of hospital personnel visiting patients in their own homes on a regular basis, providing medication where appropriate and sometimes offering support to carers. The argument in favour of home-based care is partly financial, given the assumption that it provides a less expensive alternative to hospital care (although this has been challenged (Foster *et al.*, 1991; Foster, n.d.). It partly follows, as well, from the related problem of limited hospital facilities. Advocacy of home care is also related to the nature of HIV/AIDS, which may involve a series of crises interspersed with periods of relatively good health over months or years. Chikankata not only pioneered and publicised this type of programme, but also offers training to others wishing to adapt it to their specific needs. In Zambia, some home care programmes have been run by hospitals or health centres, and others by churches or community organisations, reaching a combined total of at least 100 by 1996 (Republic of Zambia, 1997).

The need for counselling, prior and subsequent to a diagnosis for HIV or AIDS, was also perceived as a gap needing urgent attention in the first years of the epidemic. Counselling is often included as part of a home-based care package, and is also carried out by trained personnel in hospitals and health centres. A specialist Zambian NGO, Kara Counselling, was established in this area in 1989, to provide both counselling and training of counsellors. Founded by individuals associated with Lusaka's University Teaching Hospital, it was subsequently supported by a number of a number of donors including NORAD, the United States Agency for International Development (USAID), and the United Nations Children's and Education Fund (UNICEF) (Hughes-d'Aeth, 1998).

NGO activity in Tanzania appeared slightly later and would seem to be less extensive than in Zambia. There is no parallel in Tanzania to the widespread and focused anti-AIDS clubs, although there are many uncoordinated initiatives in schools and amongst youth in general. Home-based care programmes, though badly needed, have not emerged in the organised and extensive way they did in Zambia. There have nevertheless been significant and innovative achievements. One of the most important AIDS organisations in Tanzania is Walio katika Mapambano ya AIDS, Tanzania (WAMATA), discussed in detail in Chapter 8. Founded in the late 1980s, it emerged from concern to provide care and support for people with HIV and AIDS by those who had experienced the effects of the epidemic at close hand, including individuals living with HIV or AIDS. It does advocacy and educational work and is involved in counselling and care. From an initial branch in Dar es Salaam, WAMATA has extended its activities throughout several regions in the country and has added a vibrant youth section.

Also important was the donor supported programme of condom distribution, handled under the USAID funded NGO, PSI. In Tanzania subsidised condoms under the brand-name '*Salama*' (safety/peace) have been distributed to all areas of the country through 'social marketing' practices very much in keeping with neo-liberal formulas of extending the market and generating entrepreneurial activity (Baylies and Bujra, 1995). Condoms are sold on licence to 'deserving' groups or individuals who are thus enabled to accumulate in a small way. By 1998[15], more than a million *Salama* condoms were being sold every month, although this represented a levelling off after an earlier dramatic rise in the sales curve. In Zambia, where a similar operation distributes condoms under the brand name 'Maximum,' about 18 million condoms were distributed in total in 1996, with 7.4 million being sold by the condom social marketing project (Republic of Zambia, 1997).

It is difficult to say how many local and international NGOs are engaged in AIDS work in either country. In Tanzania, some such as the Scripture Union, Baraza Kuu la Waislamu Tanzania (the national Muslim Association), the Tanzanian Scouts Association and the African Medical and Research Foundation have added AIDS concerns to their existing portfolio. Some Africa-wide initiatives, like the Society for Women and AIDS in Africa, led to the formation of local branches in Tanzania and Zambia. In other cases groups appear like mushrooms and fade away within a short period as funding efforts fail. In 1997, Zambia's National AIDS Network had 339 members across the country. However, many of these were government departments, hospitals, church bodies or individual anti-AIDS clubs or home-based care programmes (ZNAN, 1997).

Strengths of collective efforts around AIDS

Action around AIDS directed at both prevention and care involves the exercise of great compassion and creative utilisation of existing expertise and organisational capacity. It often reflects a process of learning, adapting and seeking more appropriate means of effective intervention. Although local initiative and ownership have been crucial to sustainability from the beginning, collaboration has also been an important hallmark of efforts.

Introduction from early on of a wide range of educational techniques

The importance of education was seized on early in the epidemic and encouraged by external advisors on the assumption that it was ignorance which led to risky sexual behaviour and spread AIDS. In 1992, for example, the World Bank (1992: 141) recommended to the Tanzanian government that 'effective IEC (programmes conveying information, education and communication about AIDS) has been recognised as the major tool available to combat the epidemic'. IEC activities have included awareness campaigns, training of those otherwise involved in the spheres of health and education, incorporation of AIDS education in schools and development of peer education and collective learning initiatives.

AIDS education undertaken by the Copperbelt Health Education Project during its first year provides an illustration of the range of media used in awareness campaigns. As well as modifying Anti-AIDS Project literature, CHEP produced 500 sets of flip charts for use as teaching aids, 10,000 copies of a leaflet directed at adults and 5500 posters. AIDS information was disseminated through the mass media, via messages on the front pages of national newspapers, a weekly newspaper column and a five minute slot in a religious radio broadcast. Posters were displayed in public places, AIDS song and drama contests were organised and street theatre performances given, announced by drums, introduced by humorous sketches and featuring plays about AIDS which encouraged discussion by the audience (Mouli, 1991).

Drama was recognised early in the epidemic to be a crucial tool for making messages palatable and engaging audience involvement (Mwila and Chipeka, 1989). It has the capacity to reach all members of a society, whatever their place of residence or level of education and permits a collective gaze to fall on what might otherwise be hidden, often using humour to prompt critical appraisal of conventional behaviour. Other modes of communication have also been employed, including comics for children and videos for all ages. Advertisements for condoms appearing in newspapers and on hoardings have opened up a previously taboo subject. A radio soap opera, *Geuza Mwendo* (let's move with the times) has been followed weekly by some 6 million Tanzanians. Early in 1999, they tuned in anxiously to follow the fortunes of a truck driver, Mashaka, fully aware that his penchant for having a girl-friend in every town put him at risk of HIV (*Guardian*, UK, 4 January 1999). Television also featured in the mid 1990s in Zambia and later in Tanzania as a medium for opening up public discussion around otherwise delicate and difficult subjects, with quite considerable success.

AIDS training has been extended to groups who deal with health and education matters in the hope that this will improve their own practice and enlist them in the teaching or advising of others. As well as those in the formal sector, attempts have been made to liaise with and offer training to traditional healers, traditional birth attendants and traditional educators, and to integrate them into government or NGO initiatives. The importance of work with traditional healers cannot be underestimated, given the extent to which so many, especially in the rural areas, turn to their services, by choice or in the absence of adequate local medical facilities.

As late as 1998 it was admitted that a national AIDS curriculum for primary schools in Tanzania had yet to be developed (NACP, 1998a: 23). In some areas there was an active programme of educational work, linking it with community action but it was not always infused with gender awareness or an acknowledgement of the actuality of young people's sexual activities. In Zambia, anti-AIDS clubs have been situated in schools, but increasingly out-of-school youth have been targeted as well.[16] In both Zambia and Tanzania a range of peer education initiatives have been introduced as means to spread awareness of dangers of AIDS and means of protection among specific groups, whether commercial sex workers, married women, school leavers, factory workers or traders. Collective learning strategies have also been implemented via programmes such as ActionAid's *Stepping* Stones, and a package of activities produced by the Lusaka Interfaith HIV/AIDS Network-ing Group (Banda *et al.*, n.d.) – combining training in 'life skills' with more specific discussion of sexual health.

Utilisation of existing organisational capacity

Existing organisational expertise and capacity have been drawn upon, enlisting support and extending the activities of international and local NGOs. Of particular importance (although also beset with contradictions) have been the churches. In Zambia as many as 70 per cent of the population regard themselves as Christians and church networks are perhaps the most widespread and strongest within the country. Tanzania has greater religious pluralism, with approximately 44 per cent of the population regarding themselves as Christian and 33 per cent as Moslem. Local leaders of both religions are often key to opinion formation.

Within both countries, the support of local churches, their leaders and their congregations may be crucial to building and sustaining community-based AIDS initiatives.[17] In Rungwe in Tanzania, where 95 per cent of the population are Christian, Kaihula (1996) found the churches to be more important than government in provision of educational and health services. The three hospitals in the area were run, respectively, by Roman Catholics, Lutherans and Moravians and all secondary schools, save three, were run by different Christian denominations, as were several teachers colleges and technical schools. Government officials at ward level found it necessary to work closely with the churches in order to ensure that their own programmes enjoyed support and success. It was the churches in Rungwe, moreover, which operated AIDS counselling centres and provided home-based care. In Zambia, similarly, although many government hospitals have implemented home-based care programmes, these were initially promoted by mission hospitals where the underlying ethos fostered charity and compassion. These same values have been crucial to enlisting the involvement of many individuals in community work around AIDS.

Recognition of the need for networking and co-ordination

Collaboration, sharing of information and expertise and establishing partnerships have been fundamental to AIDS activities. In Zambia a plan for a National AIDS Network was germinated among delegates to a conference for AIDS NGOs held in Nairobi in 1988. The following year they set up a Co-ordinating Committee, which organised a Church Leaders' Conference and, in 1990, the first of what were to become annual national AIDS NGOs Conference (ZNAN Secretariat, 1997).[18] The changing format and content of these conferences, as well as the composition of participants within them, reveal something of the history of work around AIDS in Zambia. The first had strong representation from mission hospitals and religious organisations, including chaplaincies with the armed forces and the University Teaching Hospital. Over subsequent years representation extended to include those from local NGOs, as well as from UN bodies, the donor community and the government. The second conference, in 1991, addressed the fundamental purpose of the network through its very theme, 'Sharing the Challenge', and the opening address, by the Minister of Health, acknowledged that 'government, non-governmental organisations and all health workers should bear their share of responsibility for preventing AIDS and looking after those who are HIV positive and those who have developed AIDS' (Mudenda, 1991).[19]

In Tanzania, the degree of co-ordination and the extent of joint activities has been less and more recent. The Tanzania AIDS Project (TAP) was set up in 1993, with funding from USAID, to build the capacity of local NGOs and co-ordinate overall activity. Further co-ordination was achieved among NGOs in Dar es Salaam in conjunction with TAP in the mid 1990s with the establishment of an umbrella structure (the Dar Cluster), through which a system of referrals operates to ensure that the particular expertise of specific NGOs is effectively utilised. Some of the major national AIDS NGOs in Tanzania – African Medical Research Foundation (AMREF), WAMATA, Society for Women and AIDS in Tanzania (SWAAT) and Tanzania Gender Networking Programme (TGNP) – regularly serve as sources of advice and expertise for smaller NGOs and community-based organisations (Mbilinyi and Mwabuki, 1996).

Co-ordination and sharing of experience is not confined within national boundaries. Regular sessions of the International Conference on AIDS and STDs in Africa (ICASA) have been particularly significant, but there have been many other meetings and workshops where knowledge has been shared, such as a conference for journalists on the reporting of AIDS held in Lusaka in 1992 (Mwanza, 1993). Continental-wide NGOs are also important, not least the Society for Women and AIDS in Africa. Sharing has also occurred in other ways. WAMATA in Tanzania, for example, gained crucial advice and training from the AIDS Support Organisation (TASO) in Uganda and Chikankata Hospital's home-based care programme in Zambia before developing its own programme appropriate to the specific needs of Tanzania.[20] Zambia's anti-AIDS clubs have served as a model for programmes in Botswana, Zimbabwe and Senegal,[21] while the Anti-AIDS Project has utilised materials developed in neighbouring countries, including *Straight Talk*, a Ugandan magazine designed to inform young people about the dangers of AIDS.

While filling gaps left by government programmes, NGOs have sometimes enjoyed a mutually supportive relationship with government bodies. In Zambia, innovations emerging from within the NGO sector, such as home-based care programmes and counselling protocols have been adopted by government institutions, with considerable sharing of materials and collaborative health education work. The Copperbelt Health Education Programme emerged from work of the Copperbelt Province AIDS Surveillance Committee, which has continued to monitor the activities of AIDS-related NGOs in the province and assist them in seeking donor funds (Mudenda, 1991). From its inception, the Anti-AIDS Project worked closely with the AIDS education unit of Zambia's Ministry of Health and the Ministry of Education in developing and disseminating materials (Mwila and Chipeka, 1989). In Tanzania, WAMATA maintained close ties with hospitals as well as with the NACP.

Assistance from external agencies

Collaboration between NGOs and government has been encouraged and facilitated by external agents, including UN bodies and bilateral donors. UNDP has placed international volunteers from Africa and the Caribbean into local AIDS programmes. International organisations within the UN family have been critically important in developing models of intervention and collaboration as well as support for specific projects. Individual donors have also been significant in direct funding or in sponsoring research. Both Zambia and Tanzania have had support from the same collection of donors – principally the UK, Norway, the EU (European Union) and the US, but also Germany, the Netherlands, Sweden, Denmark and Canada. International NGOs have also played a significant role, including the Young Women's Christian Association (YWCA), Oxfam, CARE International and ActionAid.

Problems, limitations and contradictions

For all the strengths and accomplishments of AIDS programmes in Tanzania and Zambia and their development of innovative techniques and new skills, there are many problems, with continuing gaps, and extensive unmet need. Despite recognition of the importance of co-ordination, pooling of efforts and utilisation of knowledge gained from experience, there remain instances of wasteful competition, uneven geographical coverage, duplicated effort, and repetition of strategies which have elsewhere met with limited success. Despite the relative success of awareness campaigns in increasing knowledge about AIDS, encouraging more open discussion about sexual behaviour and inducing some behavioural change, progress in these areas is far too restricted and at too slow a pace given the urgency of the situation. Ideologies and orientations which have guided some partners, such as religious groups, have not always been helpful. While their assistance is critical, donor preferences have sometimes dictated a direction and substance of activities at variance with what local activists or government personnel might have preferred. Most fundamentally, problems of resourcing programmes have continued to dog efforts around AIDS and have led to the serial demise of many initiatives to the repeated frustration of both potential beneficiaries and local facilitators.

Limited national resources and contradictory impact of donor policies

Considerable external funding has been directed toward AIDS activities. The budget of the NACP in Tanzania over its first 5 years, for example, was $US 11 million (World Bank, 1992: 137). Donor support to Zambia's National

AIDS Prevention and Control Programme during the period 1988–93 was higher, at $US 20 million. Yet at $.04 per capita, the Zambian figure still represented a huge shortfall against the World Bank's recommendation of $3 per capita expenditure in respect of HIV/AIDS at this stage of the epidemic (NASTLP, 1993).

AIDS tightened its grip on Tanzania and Zambia at a point when they were firmly locked in the embrace of International Monetary Fund with its neoliberal formulas dictating that public spending be reduced, government cut down to size, and private provision encouraged. When the World Bank (1992: xxxvii) carried out its country study of the AIDS problem in Tanzania, it concluded perversely that the general medicine should be applied here as well: 'the success of the fight against AIDS will... be closely linked with the determination of Tanzania policy makers to pursue [neoliberal] economic reform...'

The consequences were predictable, with public health services being wound down and user fees introduced or increased at the very time that HIV infection was rising.[22] A Christian Aid report on Tanzania summed up the position in 1999:

> Tanzania now spends nearly four times more on servicing external debt than it does on health. Government spending on health has been cut by about 15 per cent since 1990. The number of hospital beds per patient has fallen by over one-third between 1980 and 1994. In 1996–97 the Tanzanian government health budget was only about $1.50 per head (compared with World Bank estimates of minimal required spending in low income countries of about $11.00 per head).[23]

> (www.christian-aid.org.uk)

Periodic reviews have highlighted the poverty of resources and conditions which frame AIDS health care in both countries – the lack of sterilising equipment to ensure that infections are not transmitted via hypodermic needles, the lack of bottles with which to store tested blood, the dire shortages of drugs to treat STDs or of counsellors to assist those with AIDS come to terms with their diagnoses (Hoelsher *et al.*, 1994; Lie and Biswalo 1994; Vos *et al.*, 1994; Republic of Zambia 1997).[24] And this is not even to note the non-availability of antiretrovirals which permit many in the West to live longer with AIDS, but which in Tanzania and Zambia are accessible only to the very rich, through private channels. Others are lucky to have opportunistic infections attended to with standard treatments; often they are simply sent home to die (Baylies, 1999b).

The directives and behaviour of donors and international agencies have sometimes confounded and complicated attempts to confront the threat of AIDS, while ostensibly oriented toward strengthening it. The dissolution of the Global Programme on AIDS (GPA) and the policy of decentralisation of the health sector, recommended (in truth imposed) by external monitors, can serve as two illustrations. The restructuring of AIDS related activities by members of the UN family under the rubric of UNAIDS was carried out in order to rationalise provision and promised considerable benefit. However, in the short run the removal of GPA, which had formerly funded elements of country plans not covered by other donors, left a resource gap. In Zambia, supplies of condoms and test kits were disrupted and AIDS workers left in the lurch (Republic of Zambia, 1997). The virtues of decentralisation were extolled by the World Bank to Tanzanians (1992: 152) as a means of bringing the battle against AIDS to local people. In practice, it has often dissipated and fragmented efforts. In Zambia, health sector decentralisation threatened both to isolate the national AIDS control programme, as one unit among nine under the Public Health Systems Section of the Ministry of Health, with no official links to AIDS programmes at provincial or district level, and to render attention to it at local level far more diffuse (Republic of Zambia, 1997). When the reforms worked through to the district level in Mansa in Zambia's Luapula Province, for example, the individual who had formerly been district AIDS officer was re-designated Information Officer for Health, with AIDS only one of her several responsibilities.[25]

The question of incentives or personal compensation

Problems of limited and unreliable resources in the fight against AIDS filter from national to community level, affecting both government divisions and NGOs. They underline the need for careful planning and encouragement of a spirit of volunteerism to ensure sustainability without undue dependence on donors. However, this in turn poses difficulties. Compassion and commitment are abundantly demonstrated, but the limited resources of the nation are mirrored in limited income of would-be volunteers, and repeated worries are raised about lack of incentives. Participants in a seminar representing some of the key AIDS NGOs in Tanzania stressed the tension between volunteerism and personal financial need, as well as between personal commitment and inadequate organisational resources. Enthusiasm was typically high at the beginning of activities, but waned as everyday financial difficulties intruded (Mbilinyi and Mwabuki, 1996). Similar concerns have been repeatedly raised in Zambia. As the following recommendation indicates, volunteerism is recognised as a virtue in itself and as something to be nurtured:

> While peer educators should be paid, money should never be the focus of interactions. It should be given, recognising its inadequacy, as a gratuity and the co-ordinators must emphasise peer educators' sacrifice and public spiritedness.
>
> (Chalowandya and Chitomfwa, 1995b)

Still, the need for individual livelihoods to be secured before community work can be undertaken remains pressing. As a woman in Lusaka commented, 'I used to do voluntary work but at the end of the day I got nothing from it. I am a widow. What will I feed my children with?'[26]

Frustrations about volunteerism become all the greater when the perverse way in which AIDS work has become a 'business' (Setel, 1996) for some becomes increasingly obvious. For those well-placed to take advantage, the tragedy offers new opportunities, not just for the coffin makers and the dispensers of medicine and 'cures', but also for those able to secure jobs in AIDS organisations and government facilities providing education, counselling, treatment, liaison and administration. As Seeley *et al.* (1992) found in Uganda, the mapping of rewards to a hierarchy of positions in AIDS programmes can create inequalities or exacerbate those already present, whether at community level or more widely. There is all too frequently a gender dimension to such patterns of inequality. Mbilinyi and Mwabuki's (1996) investigation of AIDS NGOs in Tanzania found an under-representation of women at top levels and over-representation among the ranks of their volunteers. The situation was similar in Zambia. In 1994, only one among the co-ordinator and deputies at the national AIDS office was female. Of major NGOs within the country in the health and population area, only a handful were headed by women (Mutepa, 1994).

Obstacles to programme sustainability

A certain cynicism attends the evaluation of some AIDS NGOs, which are seen as 'on paper' only, or devices for securing funds from donors for the pockets of their officers, or composed of a few relatively well-to-do individuals, who use them as badges of their concern. A member of an Anti-AIDS Artists group in Zambia complained that, in addition, 'a lot of funds are being spent on projects which do not bear fruit. Many people enjoy attending seminars but after these seminars, nothing is done even to impart knowledge to others' (Mudenda, 1991). In many cases, however, it is simply that what is 'on paper' and may have once been viable has faded away. Sometimes this indicates diminishing commitment, but in other cases it follows from the ending of material support or lack of means for translating training into practice.

The anti-AIDS clubs in Zambia can serve to illustrate some of the difficulties faced. By the mid 1990s almost 2000 had been registered. However, an extensive internal review revealed that many were inactive. In Kabwe district of Central Province, where an officer of the provincial office of the Ministry of Education had been appointed to co-ordinate club activities and had formed a patrons' association among local professionals, 62 per cent of local clubs were very active. But this was true of few of those elsewhere in the province. Similarly, in Southern Province's Mazabuka and Monze districts only 28 per cent were active, almost all of them initiated by Chikankata or Chikuni Mission Hospitals. Problems were often less disinterest than economic dislocation. Many schools had been reduced to skeletal staffs, with motivated club patrons among those having departed. School infrastructure was often so poor that clubs lacked accommodation. However, of particular significance was the drought, which had afflicted much of the country during the previous 3 years. In Central Province's Serenje district it had had a 'devastating' impact on school attendance, pushing 'most school going youth into risky behaviour in the search for food and funds to meet their school financial obligations' (Chalowandya and Chitomfwa, 1995a: 4). At one primary school in Southern Province teachers were trying to persuade students to stay in school by organising three meals per week: 'when you see our girls move up and down they are not looking for men. It is money. It is difficult to fight against AIDS because it is transmitted through our very fibre of existence' (Kalipenta and Chalowandya, 1995).

Problems of transport frequently figure in the ineffectiveness or demise of many groups and programmes. In Eastern Province lack of transport to permit networking among anti-AIDS clubs limited their work and the evaluation team recommended that bicycles and motor bikes should be an essential part of a rescue plan (Chalowandya and Chitomfwa, 1995). A brief tour of Zambia's Luapula Province in October 1995 as a preliminary to our research there found a number of AIDS programmes to have stalled through lack of transport.[27] In Tanzania there are similar problems. A shortage of funds for transport allowances to permit attendance at meetings, let alone for vehicles, plagues operations and leads to inactivity and demoralisation among staff.

Problems of co-ordination

Duplication of efforts, fragmentation and competition are visible on many levels and in many forms. Knowledge gained is too seldom shared and individuals and groups repeatedly re-learn lessons struggled through earlier by those in adjacent communities. A number of attempts have been made to compile bibliographies and catalogue AIDS materials, from which several useful documents have resulted, notably the *HIV/AIDS Bibliography, an annotated review of research on HIV/AIDS in Zambia* (NASTLP and UNICEF, 1996). In Tanzania, the NACP has created a library and computer listing of research publications whose entries are routinely forwarded to the Ministry of Health for information and action (NACP, 1998). However, project documentation frequently remains unavailable (sometimes unwritten) or hopelessly dispersed.

Recommendations continue to be churned out to effect greater co-ordination, while in practice relations among would-be partners are frequently strained. If the Copperbelt Health Education Project in Zambia enjoyed close relations with government at district and provincial levels, this experience was not shared by NGOs in the country's capital. (Mudenda, 1991). However, government workers also find themselves at a disadvantage. When directed to co-ordinate international and local NGO activity with state sector services in conjunction with a decentralisation directive, local government officers in Kagera in Tanzania found themselves unable to do so effectively. They were poorly informed about the extent of HIV seropositivity in the area and had far less funding than many of the NGOs whose work they were supposed to oversee: 'the lack of financial resources...placed local government in the position of having to accept any help offered' (Koekkoek and Steenbeck, 1995: 15). International NGOs in the region were less than open with government officials about their activities and often saw themselves as 'independent organisations with their own policies and objectives', for whom government should ensure an 'obstacle-free environment' (ibid.).

Local NGOs and donors have also suffered uneasy relations. Local people despair when donors do not fund administrative expenses, essential to ensuring accountability and programme success. Moreover, donors have been known to set up projects and then leave without transferring expertise so that local people could maintain them (Mudenda, 1991). Conversely donors point to NGO claims to be addressing the AIDS epidemic as a marketing instrument, a bid for external funding (Koekkoek and Steenbeck, 1995). Different donors tread on different sides of the line of variously dictating the content of projects or supporting local initiatives which seem well planned and appropriate to their stated ends. In either case there is often a professed difficulty in accurately evaluating the potential of new organisations and hence a tendency to stick with those tried and tested.[28]

Uneven geographical spread

AIDS activity in both Tanzania and Zambia is characterised by uneven spread, with large gaps in coverage, primarily in rural areas and often irrespective of the level of HIV prevalence which characterises them. The great majority of NGOs listed as members of the Zambia National AIDS Network (ZNAN) were located in Lusaka (ZNAN, 1997) and for many, their work was largely confined there. Only seven organisations are included on a list of AIDS NGOs operating in Tanga Region in Tanzania, where Lushoto is located, most of them operating from Tanga town.[29] In another part of Tanzania, Kyela district in Rungwe, with one of the highest levels of HIV prevalence in the country, NGOs had little visibility (Aggleton and Warwick, 1999). Nor, apart from the network of anti-AIDS clubs, were NGOs found to be active in AIDS work in Petauke and Nyimba districts of Zambia's Eastern Province (Chalowandya and Chitomfwa, 1995b).

Disparate agendas and the impact of underlying ideologies

The absence of NGOs, however, does not imply the absence of work around AIDS. As already noted, a considerable contribution is made by the churches. In Petauke and Nyimba districts, for example, local churches and mission hospitals had spearheaded education programmes, and organised home-based care programmes and support for orphans. For all the benefits brought by such programmes, whether under the auspices of NGOs, churches or the government, their nature and content is often slanted by the ideology of the funding or implementing body. Appropriateness of message, medium and mode of intervention are frequently determined by external judgement.

It is around the issue of prevention, ideas about causation and the apportioning of blame for AIDS that differences of approach are most evident. The Catholic church and some evangelical sects have often been antagonistic to the use of condoms, seeing this as a concession to sinful behaviour. Instead they advocate self control, expressed in abstinence before marriage and fidelity within it. Muslim leaders in Tanzania have spoken of AIDS as 'God's big stick', the deserved wages of sin. A Lutheran Bishop in Tanzania's Mbeya region, argued that the government was encouraging people to commit adultery by advocating the use of condoms. However, worst of all, from his perspective, was that children were being taught about sex and instructed in the virtues of condoms (Kaihula, 1996).

In other cases, however, those with strong Christian beliefs have conceded the need for condoms in the interests of their children's survival.[30] In Zambia the anti-AIDS clubs serve as an example of guiding principles evolving to ensure that young people have access to means of protection. Here the dominant message adopted early on – 'don't play sex! No sex before marriage' – has been subject to much reflection, leading to an increasing conviction that young people need to work out for themselves the most appropriate means of protection rather than having this dictated to them by their elders.[31] In Tanzania, something of this same transition can be traced through published research, as well as practice, where a shift in moral perspectives is evident, away from repression and towards an understanding of the dilemmas that face young people and an acceptance that they need negotiating skills as well as awareness of the value of condoms (Tumbo-Masabo and Liljestrom, 1994; Van Eeuwijk and Mlangwa, 1997).

Focus on gender and community action

As noted above, the second medium term plan in Zambia registered a shift – at least at the level of rhetoric – towards the need not just to educate for behavioural change, but to address underlying structural factors which contribute to relative vulnerability to HIV. At the same time in both countries the importance of facilitating community-based programmes was affirmed. How far has such a shift, reflecting broader trends in global AIDS programmes, been registered in practice across both countries? To what extent has there been increased emphasis on women, and more importantly, how far have *gender* relations been brought into view? To what extent and in what way have communities been supported?

Evidence of gender awareness?

The position of women as carers, widows and people living with HIV and AIDS has been the subject of research commissioned by Zambia's AIDS control programme (Mulenga, 1993; Macwan'gi *et al.*, 1994) or has otherwise been the subject of published studies (Mwale and Burnard, 1992; Campbell and Kelly, 1995). Gender has also been raised obliquely through discourse of 'high risk groups' where women figure large as bargirls and prostitutes in Tanzania (Nyamuryekung'e, 1996; Mgalla and Pool, 1997) or in risk environments, as in Mushingeh *et al.*'s (1990–91) account of sexual networking in the fish trade between Luapula and Zambia's Copperbelt.

A few studies in Tanzania have raised the issue of gender through considering male behaviour. From analysis of a national survey of sexual behaviour, Kapiga (1996: 441), for example, concludes that since 'high risk sexual behaviour was more common in men than in women... men may be an important source of spread of HIV infection in Tanzania' thereby justifying the targeting of men. Official acknowledgement of the need for interventions targeted at men has been justified in Tanzania as follows: 'although men and women are equally involved in unprotected multiple sexual intercourse, men have generally been responsible for initiating such risk behaviour'' (NACP, 1998a: 31). The interventions envisaged, however, targeted atypical men – truck drivers, travellers and soldiers – rather than men in general. Some studies have suggested that men are beginning to cut down on the number of sexual partners they have in response to the threat of AIDS (Ng'weshemi *et al.*, 1996). An alternative response to risk would be increased use of condoms, but more than one study has shown that condom use is very low in Tanzania (Mnyika *et al.*, 1995a,b; Kapiga, 1996) and that men dislike condoms (Setel, 1996) while women are not powerful enough to demand their use.

In both Tanzania and Zambia, 'culture' has been held up as male dominated and cultural practices as putting women particularly at risk. Mutepa (1994) refers to the way in which traditional sayings in Zambia often denigrate the position of women or women's sexuality, although Rweyemamu (1999) claims that changes in attitude are beginning to appear among young people in Tanzania. Various positions have been taken as to which sex is more likely to be blamed for the spread of HIV. Setel (1996: 1175) argues that in Kilimanjaro 'men are equally, if not more, vilified than women'. This challenges previous accounts which report women, and particularly young women being held to deserve blame for their mercenary and instrumental attitudes towards men (Hartwig, 1991; Weiss, 1993). Not simply blame but violence against women has been highlighted by others in response to men's fear of loss of control over women (Rweyemamu, 1999).

What is particularly characteristic of the literature is a unidimensional view of 'women', with a distorting focus on those assumed to be 'high risk groups'. The situation for the majority of women, whose risk derives from sex with their husbands, is infrequently addressed, nor are the dynamics of gender relations examined (Baylies and Bujra, 1995).

The argument that women are placed in a disadvantageous position in the face of AIDS by cultural practices and by their economic dependence on men is explicit in official documents and is broadcast through the media, but this insight rarely translates into official programmes, NGO activity or project work. If anything, there is a continuing tendency to focus on women rather than on gender relations and, in spite of apparently adopting a gender discourse, to continue to treat women as merely victims. Concern with structural bases for vulnerability has led to initiatives promoting income generation for widows or 'rehabilitation' of sex workers, and the need to ensure the education of girls as a means to forestall the epidemic has been recently highlighted (Republic of Zambia, 1997). However, it is rare for a link to be drawn in practice between income security and the ability of women to ensure protection against HIV, or to address the relationship between unequal power relations in public and private spheres. Tanzania's third medium term plan (NACP, 1998a: 19) asserts that the promotion of income-generating activities amongst sex workers 'empowers them to negotiate for safer sex', but there has been little attempt to assess the validity of the hypothesis that greater income security yields greater protection.

Programmes aimed at income generation or education remain a minor aspect of AIDS activity aimed at women, which in turn is but a minor element within the wider arena of AIDS programmes. Of those NGOs listed by Msaky and Kisesa (1997) as involved in AIDS related work in Dar es Salaam, the main focus was in preventive work with youth, with only a minority having any major concern for women or gender issues. The exceptions, however, are important. Among them is the local branch of the Society for Women and AIDS in Tanzania (SWAAT). It serves more than three hundred families through individual and group counselling and the provision of medicines. SWAAT, which has twenty-five branches throughout Tanzania, does not restrict its help to women, but includes their families, as well as reaching out to educate the general public through open air meetings with speakers and rap bands. Its sister organisation in Zambia, the Society for Women and AIDS in Zambia (SWAAZ) has fewer branches but still performs a crucial function, not least of publicising the specific situation of women in respect of the AIDS epidemic. A former head was subsequently appointed Minister of Health. Other NGOs concerned with women's or gender issues have added on AIDS concerns, among them the YWCA, Zambia Association for Research and Development (ZARD), Women in Law and Development in Zambia (WILDAF), Tanzania Gender Networking Programme (TGNP) and Tanzania Media Women's Association (TAMWA). The Zambian NGO, Tasintha, was formed specifically for, and to publicise the situation of, sex workers in the context of AIDS.

This listing underestimates the incorporation of gender issues – and gender awareness – in a number of other NGOs such as WAMATA in Tanzania, as well as the contribution which women have made to AIDS-related work. Women are the footsoldiers of such activity, disproportionately represented among volunteers, whether in anti-AIDS clubs, home-based care programmes or peer education. But, they are underrepresented in salaried posts, as members of review teams and among the ranks of those making policy on AIDS.

Support for community-based actions around AIDS

Community-based activity has been affirmed in official policy documents as necessary and crucial to the fight against AIDS, given limited resources and capacity of central governments. The logic in favour of more widespread participation, greater inclusiveness and indeed greater democratisation may be implicit in the very nature of the AIDS epidemic itself. As Cohen (1998a) has argued, although this societal crisis frequently elicits denial and initially repressive responses, it has the capacity to engender greater openness. By creating dilemmas which cut across class and interest group solidarity and threaten development, it *necessitates* the involvement of existing networks within, but also co-operation across, countries, potentially leading to greater justice and equity. In his words:

> While policy and programme responses in the region have initially repre-
> sented a retreat from the inclusive principles of SHD (sustainable human
> development), in some countries there is now a gradual realisation that an
> effective response requires the active participation of civil society. Para-
> doxically the HIV epidemic has created a need and an opportunity for
> innovative approaches to governance, which make the processes needed
> for SHD more attainable rather than less so.
>
> (Cohen, 1998a)

Cohen acknowledges the large gap which remains between this possibility and present reality. The new role of the state in relation to civil society which he envisions, emergent at least in part from the AIDS crisis, would appear still far from being realised in the cases of Tanzania and Zambia. There are glimmers of it in rhetorical gestures of support for community-based action, but doubts have been expressed as to how far leaders fully grasp the enormity of the epidemic's impact, given their tendency to seek normalisation by persistently treating AIDS as primarily a health problem (Republic of Zambia, 1997: 33; NACP, 1998a).

Assuming ownership of the epidemic at the highest level has been repeat-edly called for. In both countries political leaders have made public declara-tions of commitment to the fight against AIDS. The former President of Zambia addressed the Fifth International Conference on AIDS in 1989 (Schoepf, 1991) and his admission that one of his sons had died from AIDS was highly significant in opening the subject to more public view. At the 6th National AIDS Conference in Zambia in 1996 a message was read on behalf of his successor, President Chiluba, declaring that 'our nation is at war with AIDS'. In this same year the government set up a national HIV/AIDS co-ordinating committee reporting directly to the Vice President[32] and in 2000 established a National AIDS Council and Secretariat, to be supervised by a committee of Ministers.[33] In Tanzania, President Mkapa spoke out publicly about the AIDS epidemic for the first time in 1999 on the occasion of an Interministerial Technical Committee being set up (UNAIDS, 1999f).

Yet formal support has not always been matched by the structure of funding or mechanisms to facilitate the co-ordination of AIDS work. The hosting of the 11th International Conference on AIDS and STDs in Africa in Lusaka, in September 1999, served as a important occasion for highlighting issues around AIDS in Zambia, as well as an opportunity for reaffirming commit-ment by the Zambian government. However, heads of state were absent from the event itself, whether from Zambia or neighbouring countries, in marked contrast to the way in which the presence of many had graced a meeting in Libya the previous week on the (dubious) prospect of establishing a united states of Africa.

What, then, can be said about support for those involved in AIDS work at community level? Efforts have been made in both countries and there is much on the ground, but it is far less than required and many feel stranded. Telling comments appear in the 1997 review of Zambia's second medium term plan. While noting that HIV/AIDS activities ranging from IEC to home care were 'being implemented by communities themselves through anti-AIDS clubs and neighbourhood committees', sometimes with the assistance of churches and NGOs, it was also pointed out that: 'other than a few well known NGOs, most activities are home grown and under-funded. In many communities, people are sacrificing their families and time to take care of AIDS patients without recognition or support from the health system' (Republic of Zambia, 1997: 32). Many women's groups were acknowledged to be active in promot-ing safer sexual behaviour. Furthermore, 'in recognition of the burden on women and in particular on widowed women, NGO activities and activities sponsored by collaborators in the UN system, have resulted in income gener-ating activities, women's groups, support systems and direct economic support from church organisations to affected families'. But it acknowledged that these were limited in scope (ibid.: 12).

Taking seriously the need to take gender on board and promote community level activity

AIDS threatens the developmental prospects of countries such as Tanzania and Zambia, but also opens the way – of necessity – for changes in govern-ance via greater inclusiveness, which can make sustainable human develop-ment more attainable. The spread of AIDS is bound up in the inequalities of current gender relations, making women particularly vulnerable. To the degree that strategies for its containment tackle these inequalities, however, they can also contribute towards a transformation in gender relations. As argued in Chapter 1, women's networks and organising capabilities constitute an important resource in the fight against AIDS. In turn their collective action can strengthen their ability to negotiate for greater personal safety. Sustaining such efforts, however, may require women's economic security to be addressed, pointing to an intrinsic connection between protection achieved within the private sphere and women's position within the public political economy.

Governments must depend on communities helping themselves, given limited capacity and meagre state resources, and, moreover, because local level activity may in practice be more effective. However, there must be mechanisms for co-ordinating and supporting those efforts. This is not solely the responsibility of national governments. On ethical and moral grounds, assistance is required from the global community (Baylies, 1999a).

Our study has sought to take seriously claims made about gender and community action in respect of AIDS, but to treat these as matters for investigation rather than as givens. With an initial, but not exclusive, focus on women, we have sought to examine both the obstacles which block their capacity to protect themselves from AIDS and the strengths and accumulated experience which they can bring to such endeavours. From the beginning these were viewed not just as matters of theoretical interest but ones of practical urgency. It was accepted that AIDS represented a critical emergency and that research, while necessarily rigorous in its design and execution, must be oriented toward action, so far as possible.

Appendix

Methodology matters: research process and sites of study

There are a number of key areas where difficult decisions are required in designing social research on AIDS, not least as regards the ethics of intrusion in sensitive areas and the devising of means for securing reliable information. Research on a topic relating to the most private domain of social relations (sexuality and sexual relations) immediately raises issues regarding access to data and questions about its quality. Approaches which depend on direct observation and participation are generally ruled out,[34] although it is possible to draw on accounts of those who are directly affected. However, reliance on what people say about sexual activity, whether by way of individual responses to a questionnaire or in group discussions, is subject to all of the usual caveats about interviewer effects, all the more so in an area where shame or bravado often lead to economies with the truth.

There may be particular problems with survey techniques in this area, given that people's memories and forms of mental recording may not coincide with those of researchers, but also because the world of meaning and interpretation is ignored if surveys are used in isolation. What does the word 'partner' or 'sexual intercourse' mean to respondents? Would a rape victim or a child count as 'partner'? Does 'sex' include non-penetrative forms of intimacy or anal intercourse? Reliance on data from such instruments, moreover, fails to concede that people's responses are simply claims and not objective accounts of the truth.[35]

Official records and statistics of the progress of the AIDS epidemic must also be treated with the greatest caution. As we observed at first hand, their modes of production leave much to be desired and often introduce unacknowledged distortions. The uneven supply of reagents and their total absence in some health units means that precise diagnosis is made only in a small proportion of cases and many AIDS cases go unrecorded, even where doctors are fairly certain of what they see before them (Republic of Zambia, 1997).[36] Sentinel surveillance testing is often done with care but coverage is patchy year on year, making comparisons across time and place problematic. Prevalence estimates emerging from the data, and finding their way into country and UNAIDS' documentation, utilise models based on carefully considered assumptions. But these can be faulty.

Due to the limited nature of official data and the limitations of surveys for generating rich social analytical data, the research on which this volume is based combined quantitative with qualitative methodologies. The latter use 'naturalistic' methods as far as possible in an endeavour to uncover and explore the range of possible behaviours and their meanings. They seek to investigate how meanings are constructed and negotiated and how they are framed in specific social contexts. Our investigation drew (though not uncritically) on existing official and unofficial statistics where these were available, and included a small ($N = 100$) base-line survey in each of the six localities where we worked, which generated additional quantifiable material. However, it also entailed the collection of a variety of qualitative data culled from observation, participation in community activities and ceremonial occasions, key informant interviews, responses to open-ended questions in the base-line surveys, extended discussions with individuals and groups and overheard conversations. In addition, contextualising the views of speakers in respect of their social location necessitated mapping of local power structures and resource distribution as well as documenting and observing the operations of local health facilities and other relevant institutions.

The research design

Our research was carried out through two phases in six separate sites within two countries. The active period of field-work stretched over 1995 and 1996, with periodic follow-up visits to some of the sites extending through September 1999. The first phase involved analysis of the progress of the epidemic and responses to it at national level and, in each site, an initial exploration of how it was being locally experienced, understood and confronted. The second phase, with a more deliberate action orientation, involved the facilitation and monitoring of ongoing community action around AIDS, with particular attention to its gender dimensions. The project involved collaboration in the design, but particularly in its implementation, between researchers based in the UK, Tanzania and Zambia, organised in two 'country teams'.

In each country a neighbourhood within or adjacent to the capital city was chosen as one of the three sites for local in-depth research, with the others selected to illustrate contrasting perspectives on the progress of the epidemic and the extent and nature of AIDS-related activity. The multi-site, two-country design was utilised to assist an identification of both common features of the epidemic's progress and those more specific to a given context. It was intended to facilitate analysis of how AIDS intrudes into but also illuminates the particular characteristics of communities.

As our central concern was with how AIDS had impacted on and been informed by gender relations, research in each of the six sites involved an initial assessment of the prevailing relations between men and women, as well as an attempt to gain a feel for how much people knew about AIDS and how they felt it had affected the community and themselves as individuals. Given that any simple contrast between men and women could well be fractured along lines of other social divisions, we investigated these as well, giving particular attention to differentials on the basis of age and socio-economic position. In each locality our base-line survey utilised a sampling protocol entailing an equal number of males and females falling into three age categories (15–19, 20–45 and 46 and above) and three income categories.[37] These were followed by focus group discussions with groups of men and women (generally separately but occasionally mixed) in the different age categories in order to explore some of the same material in a context which permitted contrasting views to be offered and reflected upon.

Our initial hypothesis put much weight on a view of women as active citizens possessing organisational skills, which might be built upon in campaigns against HIV infection. The investigation of how far this applied required an understanding of the existing forms of collective activity amongst women in the neighbourhoods researched. In the second, more action-oriented phase of the research we shifted our focus towards a critical assessment of the way in which such skills or organisation were presently being exploited within AIDS work and, in some cases, exploration of the ways in which they might be better harnessed to this effort.

Investigation of women's sexual and health concerns and their collective action around them was complemented by research into the constraints which men put upon them in this area, as well as men's own concerns and fears. If men were alienated or ignored, then women's heightened awareness or knowledge could not be fully acted upon, since it was essentially gender *relations* which were at issue. 'Taking men on board' was assumed as crucial if women's – and men's – well-being was to be advanced. But, precisely how this might work out in practice was part of our concern – and without making the assumption that 'men' and 'masculinity' are undifferentiated categories.

Modification of the design

Designs which appear in advance to effectively translate theoretical questions into a workable formula for empirical investigation do not always work out fully in practice. Unexpected events, the fickle intervention of the 'human factor', or realisation that what appeared initially feasible is impractical or does not take into account newly discovered factors of importance may all require some adjustments. Most research projects suffer slippage between design and implementation and ours was no exception. However, in some respects this was a positive feature of the process. A series of workshops was built into the research programme to permit collective reflection by the research teams and, in some cases, consideration of the views of a wider group of academics, activists and policy makers. In consequence of these and other factors, some changes were made. One of the most significant was the expansion of the teams themselves, bringing in a number of individuals who were or had been actively involved in AIDS work. A second was a more explicit incorporation of generational differences, with more attention on young people and patterns of tension and creative engagement across generational lines.

Caveats and qualifications

Managing a research project across two countries and six sites entailed formidable problems of communication, which were not always fully surmounted. However, the design facilitated a productive sharing of knowledge, experience and new findings. This operated on a formal basis through the workshops, but the research diaries which all members kept also served as sources of individual and collective inspiration. The nature of the teams themselves, by virtue of incorporating both academics and activists, permitted the exchange of expertise and a mutual learning process. However, their composition also introduced some difficulties, particularly when a given technique was viewed differently by different team members. A case in point was the group discussion, which was variously viewed as a means for mobilisation and awareness raising or as a tool for observing the negotiation and construction of meaning.

This raises a broader point about the comparability and validity of data collected through this and other techniques and the question of what can be taken as evidence. In general our concern was to identify points of tension and contradiction and gain a grip on how the link between gender relations and AIDS was interpreted and reinterpreted and how people were coming to terms with the danger the epidemic implied for themselves and their families. In interpreting the data, we cite comments of survey respondents, provide excerpts from focus groups or offer segments of research diaries, not as the 'truth' but as windows on the dilemmas thrown up by AIDS and the way they are thought about and experienced.

For a variety of reasons the original research design was not fully implemented – or did not develop as far or in the same way – in all of the six local sites. This applied especially to the second phase of the research which was developed much further and monitored over a longer period in some cases than in others. The specific form taken by this second phase also differed depending on the extent to which there was already a 'local history' of AIDS initiatives. In some cases where members of the research team were already involved locally as activists, it sometimes proved difficult to gain sufficient distance for a critical evaluation.

Where new AIDS initiatives materialised, in part through the research itself, other dilemmas emerged, associated with the intertwining of research ethics, research objectives and the prerequisites of project feasibility. Having rejected a detached and uninvolved approach, a (partial) contradiction could still emerge between the researcher as facilitator of local action and as observer of the strengths and weaknesses which characterised it. This proved to be especially so when the very success and sustainability of an initiative depended on the availability of resources whose origin was not immediately obvious. The role of the researcher as an apparently benevolent but 'resourceless' observer could then be held up to scrutiny, along with the assumption apparently underlying the research that people at local level should be expected to practise self-help and avoid dependence on external agents. On the other hand, undertaking a role of facilitating contacts with those better endowed, liaising between a community group and people in offices, offering advice to a group, or even providing rudimentary training in the writing of proposals, minutes, budgets or agendas could verge on meddling or raising hopes (even if unintentionally), which could prove unrealistic or unachievable. The boundaries between research, mobilisation, facilitation, guidance and interference may sometimes blur. While the dictum that research should do no harm to research subjects may be adhered to, it is also important to ensure that 'action research' does not promise what it cannot deliver, thereby leaving frustration, disappointment and disinclination to participate, rather than insight, as its legacy.

Introducing the individual studies

The three research sites in Zambia were Kanyama, a suburb of the capital, Lusaka; Kapulanga, a squatter area adjacent to Mongu, the capital of Western Province; and the catchment area of a health clinic in Mansa, the capital of Luapula Province. In Tanzania, several neighbourhoods in and around Dar es Salaam constituted the first of the sites. The second was a rural area in the mountains above Lushoto in the Tanga region and the third a set of villages near Rungwe in the Mbeya region (see map).

The accounts of the six sites which follow each focus on a critical aspect of the research questions which guided the project, some drawing more on the first phase and others on the second phase. The chapters on Rungwe and Kapulanga locate the experience of AIDS in a specific historical context and in respect of the ongoing process of social change. These chapters, along with that dealing with Kanyama, explore the way AIDS is understood and how (changing) gender relations are implicated in interpretations of who is to blame and who is at risk. The chapters on Lushoto, Mansa and Kanyama address organisational initiatives around AIDS at the local level. That on Kanyama considers the problems of co-ordinating efforts within a given community, while those on Mansa and Lushoto give closer consideration to the way in which survival strategies are bound up with AIDS work. The Lushoto study examines the interplay between generation and gender, while the chapter on Mansa gives particular attention to the dynamics and characteristics of groups which make some 'work' better than others. The chapter on Dar es Salaam shifts from community to national level in analysing the work of a prominent AIDS NGO located there, WAMATA. Both this chapter and that on Mansa consider the extent to which collective efforts around AIDS impact on participants in gendered ways.

As well as variously focusing on the questions which guided the main phases of the project, the individual chapters also pick up on a set of additional themes, which serve to distinguish the experience of AIDS in the various locales from one another. One is the importance of religion, which is addressed most fully in chapters on Rungwe and Kanyama. A second is the prevalence of AIDS. Relative to national prevalence figures, most of the sites represent high (Kanyama and Rungwe) and moderately high prevalence (Kapulanga, Mansa and Dar es Salaam). The exception is Lushoto where prevalence is relatively low. A third is variability along an urban–rural dimension. Both Lushoto and Rungwe are rural sites. Kapulanga is a peri-urban settlement while the Mansa site includes both a neighbourhood on the edge of a small town and a cluster of villages adjacent to it. Kanyama in Lusaka and Dar es Salaam represent metropolitan settings.

A fourth theme is proximity to actual or potential services in respect of AIDS prevention and care – or the extent to which there have been AIDS interventions in the locality. Lushoto and Kapulanga are communities in which little AIDS activity was in evidence, while both in Mansa and Rungwe there had been interventions by churches, NGOs or donors. Kanyama represents a case of relatively high level of intervention, but also proximity to government, donor and NGO offices. The Dar study is, of course, of a national NGO. Finally, the cases vary in terms of the relative homogeneity of the population, with those of Kapulanga, Lushoto and Rungwe being relatively homogeneous and stable (albeit with experience of residents migrating out and returning). Mansa is relatively homogeneous linguistically but with many relatively recent arrivals. Dar es Salaam and Kanyama have many recent migrants among their populations and are ethnically heterogeneous, but the former is far more linguistically homogeneous than the latter.

These various dimensions of difference and specificity (as well as commonality) will be highlighted in the chapters which follow. Taken together the case studies illuminate the depth of the problem, the range of its social dimensions and the potential for progress in campaigns of protection against AIDS.

Notes

1   World Bank tables show 68 per cent of Zambia's population to have been below the poverty line in 1991 as against 51.5 per cent in Tanzania, with both figures unacceptably high. Eighty-eight per cent of Zambia's rural population was living below the poverty line at this time (World Bank, 1998). However, notions of poverty used here are relative and the figures must be treated with caution.

2   At 8.6 per cent over the period 1970–95, Tanzania's urban population annual growth rate was one of the highest among developing countries. The rate in Zambia for the period was 4.1 per cent (UNDP, 1998), Zambia's urban growth having occurred earlier in connection with the growth of the copper industry during the colonial and early post-independence periods.

3   Dates of first diagnosis in Zambia differ from one source to another. The date 1984 is given in Fylkesnes *et al.* (1994); Mukonde (1992) also gives this as the year when there was 'conclusive evidence that AIDS was present within the country'. However, others give a date of 1985 (NASTLP, 1994; Republic of Zambia, 1997; UNAIDS, 1998e).

4   Bayley (1984) reported the appearance in 1983 of a number of individuals with atypical Kaposi's sarcoma who did not respond to routine therapy and seemed to have other features similar to AIDS patients in the US.

5   While broadly indicative of the depth of the crisis, such figures, as with all estimates, need to be treated with caution.

6   Focus group, Mansa; older men, 5.96; facilitator, T. Chabala.

7   Tanzania began collecting sentinel surveillance data from ante-natal clinics in 1988, but coverage has been patchy with relatively few sites having continuous data across subsequent years. In Zambia, individual hospitals collected some data earlier, but the first national round of surveying women attending selected ante-natal clinics did not commence until 1990. New sites were added, particularly in 1994, but thereafter surveying has been sporadic.

8   The summary here is based on NACP annual reports for the late 1990s and material included in UNAIDS epidemiological fact sheet for the country. There are some shifts over the years in terms of the ranking order of regions, whether in terms of AIDS cases or HIV prevalence. NACP (1998b: 24) statistics offer qualified support for there having been a levelling-off of infection in Kagera, especially among younger women.

9   Specific figures were Livingstone, 23.8 per cent; Chelstone, 21.7 per cent; Chilenje, 29.4 per cent; Matero, 24.8 per cent; Ndola, 21 per cent (NASTLP, n.d.).

10 In recognition that those suffering from STDs run a greater risk of contracting HIV, the programme included a component to diagnose STDs at an early stage and provide clear information to those infected about HIV prevention.

11 See Baylies (1999a) for a fuller critique of the implications of this call for communities to help themselves.

12 This date is extrapolated from the comment in 1989 by Dr C. Baker who was closely involved with the Anti-AIDS Project that it had begun 3 years previously (Mwila and

Chipeka, 1989). An officer of the Family Health Trust, under which the clubs were subsequently co-ordinated gave the date as 1987 (interview, 23 November 1994).

13   Interview, Lusaka, 10 October 1994.

14   Interview, Lusaka, 23 November 1994.

15   Personal communication to J. Bujra.

16   Interview, Lusaka, 23 November 1994.

17   Several AIDS activists affirmed the need (and their practice) of contacting leaders of local churches as part of the groundwork for setting up local AIDS programmes in peer education (interviews, Lusaka, 16 November 1994; 25 November 1994).

18   These annual meetings lapsed in 1998 and 1999 when efforts were directed at orga-nising the XIth International Conference on AIDS and STDs in Africa, which was held in Lusaka, in September 1999.

19   In recognition of the need to strengthen its activities, the NGOs Co-ordinating Committee transformed itself into an independent NGO, the Zambia National AIDS Network, in 1994 (ZNAN, 1997).

20   Interview, November 1999.

21   Interview, Dar es Salaam, 23 November 1994.

22   Analysis of the impact of structural adjustment on the health sector in Tanzania, and particularly its gendered aspect, can be found in Mbilinyi (1994), Kiwara (1994) and Lugalla (1995).

23   Quoted in Britain–Tanzania Newsletter, (May, 1999) 2119, from Christian Aid's web site: http://www.christian-aid.org.uk.

24   One example brings the message home: 'the most common (needle sterilisation) equipment is an aluminium pot heated by kerosene, charcoal or even firewood' (Hoelscher *et al.*, 1994: 1610). Tibaijuka also reports another aspect of structural adjustment in the health sector – the squeeze on the wages of health workers to a sub-economic level. In Dar es Salaam (1997:965) this had led nurses to boil old syringes so that they could appropriate new disposable needles for sale.

25   Interview, Mansa, 10 September 1999.

26   Kanyama focus group, Resident Development Committee, 9.96, facilitator F. Mkan-dawire.

27   Research diary, C. Baylies. Luapula, October 1995; November, 1995.

28   Interviews, Lusaka, 1 November 1994; 21 July 1994.

29   Not listed, but an innovative group nevertheless, is the Tanga AIDS Group, whose major focus has been the linking of medical personnel with traditional healers in order to foster mutual learning (Scheinman and Mberesero, 1999).

30   See, for example, Banda *et al.* (n.d.).

31   Interview, Lusaka, 23 November 1994.

32   Text of speech of Mr Mubanga, Permanent Secretary, Luapula Province, 2 December 1996, Mansa Central Market.

33   This was intended to monitor STDs and TB as well as AIDS. See 'Zambia National AIDS Council and Secretariat' Health L. Online posting, available e-mail: health-1@hivnet.ch; 21 March 2000).

34   For a methodological review see Boulton (1994) and Wight and Bernard (1993). The problem was described in a slightly different context by a peer educator in Zambia's Southern Province who commented that distributing condoms was one thing but what actually happens to the condoms is 'too bedroom to know' (Kalipenta and Chalo-wandya, 1995).

35   Checking out how far claims have been 'adjusted' requires an investigation of actual behaviour in context, but in fact many studies utilising survey techniques do not investigate actual behaviour at all, nor devise 'triangulating' methods to cross-check their data.

36   Aggleton and Warwick (1999) comment on the unavailability of diagnostic tests in the communities studied in Kyela district of Tanzania. Inspection of hospital records

in Luapula and interviews with health workers there confirm the sporadic supply of test kits and of the official recording of AIDS cases or mortality due to AIDS. (Mansa Hospital records 1995; interview 21 November 1995).

37 The sampling rubric used was as follows:

Socio-economic status	Female			Male		
	15–19 years	*20–45 years*	*46+ years*	*15–19 years*	*25–45 years*	*46+ years*
High	2	3	2	2	3	2
Middle	4	12	4	4	12	4
Low	5	14	4	5	14	4

3 AIDS in Kapulanga, Mongu: poverty, neglect and gendered patterns of blame

Ann Sikwibele, Caroline Shonga and
Carolyn Baylies

Introduction

> People fear AIDS because it is everywhere and has come to stay and because it kills.
> People fear death, many have died.
> Not only this village, it's world-wide.[1]

(Kapulanga survey respondents)

With reference to Kapulanga, a squatter settlement on the outskirts of Mongu in Zambia's Western Province, this chapter examines the way responses to AIDS are influenced by cultural background and historical experience.[2] Situated on the edge of the flood plain of the Zambezi river and the capital of Zambia's Western Province, Mongu is an important commercial and administrative centre. But at a distance some 600 kilometres to the west of Lusaka, it is far from the heart of Zambia's urban corridor, nor it is on an international border, nor even on a transnational road network. The tarmac road, which leads to the town, was in a state of disrepair during much of the 1990s, making travel difficult and travel times unpredictable. Although the Zambezi river forms an important conduit of transport and trade, its floodwaters also cut the town off from the western part of the province, and Angola beyond it, for several months each year. Yet in spite of this apparent context of relative isolation, AIDS is deeply entrenched in the town and its suburbs. According to national estimates (Ministry of Health, Zambia, 1997), as many as a quarter of Mongu's adult population were infected with HIV in 1997, marginally fewer than the urban prevalence in that year in several of Zambia's other provinces, but still a deeply disturbing figure.

Although the experience of AIDS in Kapulanga bears similarity to that in other parts of Zambia, its specific nature has been shaped by local cultural understandings and historical patterns of integration within a wider political economy. AIDS has been incorporated into the complex of problems people face in this locality with something of the same ambivalence which characterises their broader experiences with the contemporary Zambian state. The conviction that something must be done jostles with a sense of being neglected and unsupported. Even if believing AIDS to have been brought from outside, members of the community acknowledge that it 'has come to stay' and that its local spread is firmly grounded in the material and social conditions of the present – in local behaviour and local poverty. When seeking to come to terms with it, however, they draw on deep-seated cultural beliefs stretching back to the past. On this basis, a tendency to interpret social change through a gender lens, and to regard women's behaviour as disproportionately responsible for moral decline, has had implications for the way in which blame is apportioned.

Western Province as the former Barotseland: proud past, uncertain future

The political history of Western Province is unique within Zambia, given the relative political autonomy it enjoyed as Barotseland or Bulozi, the place of the Lozi people, throughout the colonial period. Coming from the north, the Lozi settled several centuries ago on the floodplain of the upper Zambezi, subordinating the existing population and establishing an intricately structured, centralised system, headed by a king (the Litunga). The geographical focus of Bulozi and the locus of internal trade and production was the Zambezi river. Its annual flooding across the vast expanse of the plain entailed a seasonal pattern of movement, most graphically symbolised in the ritual shifting of the Litunga's residence each spring from the floodplain to its margins, and his return each summer.

The Lozi kingdom was caught up in larger pretensions of conquest and expansion in the Southern African region when it suffered temporary subordination to a Basuto group, the Kololo, in the middle years of the nineteenth century. Much later in the century – amidst a turbulent political and economic reordering of the region – the leadership of a reconsolidated Lozi state sought to construct a path towards a viable future (Ranger, 1965; Prins, 1980). Their objective was to drive a bargain securing economic advantage, preservation of cultural and political integrity and protection against threatened incursion by the Ndebele to their south-east.

Reading the signs and sifting alternatives, the Litunga sought protectorate status from the British. When he signed the Lochnar Agreement in 1890, however, it was not with the British Crown as he imagined, but with agents of the British South Africa Company (Hall, 1965; Caplan, 1970; Mainga, 1973). In exchange for rights to explore for and extract minerals across the whole of what was to become Northern Rhodesia (to which the Lozi made exaggerated claim), the company offered protection against outside interference and attack, an undertaking not to interfere with the king's authority over his subjects, and annual payments to the king and councillors. Several months later, amidst local grumbling that his signature amounted to 'selling the country', the king attempted to renounce the treaty (Mainga, 1973). While insisting on its validity, the company, for its part, proceeded to renege on many of the commitments it embodied (Caplan, 1970).

Still, a special status *was* negotiated which set Barotseland apart and some benefits were exacted for the local population. The Lozi's apparent early victory in gaining 'permission' to retain a large degree of local administrative control, however, set in train a line of tension with the larger colony and, subsequently, with the Zambian state, which has not always worked to local advantage. Its special status brought the Lozi establishment into conflict, for example, with elements of the nationalist movements which overthrew colonialism. Although the Barotseland Agreement, signed on the eve of independence in 1964, formally recognised the Litunga as the principal local authority in Barotseland, it was rapidly undermined by the new government via a series of new acts.

Questions of allegiance and relative autonomy have marked out the political space since independence and continue to the present, with the Lozi ruling elite taking its grievances to court at the end of the twentieth century, intent on restoring the abrogated agreement. Tensions have been fuelled throughout this time by periodic claims that the national government has neglected the developmental and social service needs of the province (Gertzel, 1984). According to a survey of the local electorate in the province conducted just prior to Zambia's parliamentary and presidential elections in 1996, for example, 78 per cent rated the national government's performance in the province, 'poor' or 'very poor'. At the same time, almost 80 per cent rated their belief in traditional issues and authority as strong or very strong (Sumbwa, 1996).

The situation of Barotseland has long been characterised by a combination of insular and outward engaging tendencies. Young Lozi men trekked to find work in the South African diamond fields as early as the 1880s (Hall, 1965). In the 1930–40s, when well established recruitment agencies sent thousands annually to South African mines, over half of the male labour force of Mongu District was designated as 'absentee' (Pim and Milligan, 1938). The early provision of schools meant exporting educated individuals (mainly men, but later women as well) who made up disproportionate numbers, first of civil servants and later of professionals, in the country's line-of-rail towns. However, while there was outward movement, there was relatively little movement into the province by others from the territory and, later, the independent state. Lozi remains a language which few non-Lozi speak and though Zambia has long had a practice of civil servants being posted across the country, there has been less mixing of groups in Western Province than elsewhere.

These points set the general historical and political context in terms of which the AIDS epidemic entered the province. We now review the experience of that epidemic by residents of Kapulanga, on the edges of Mongu, using data from our baseline survey there in 1996, supplemented by data from Zambia's *Demographic and Health Survey 1996* (Central Statistical Office, Zambia, 1997), to build a picture of the lives of community members. Particular attention is given to the economic and health environment and to the pattern of gender relations which informs social interaction.

Kapulanga: getting by with difficulty

Kapulanga is one of several squatter areas on the outskirts of Mongu. Located a few kilometres from the town, its very first resident was a worker with the roads department, who, in the absence of alternative accommodation, established his home there in 1962. When several other families joined him from a residential area in the middle of Mongu, the small community was born. Its numbers expanded when residents of a squatter settlement next to the town's mortuary were sent there in 1966, and over the following 3 years, as refugees fleeing political dislocation in Angola moved in. Others have come after retirement, on losing housing previously connected with their employment. By the mid 1990s, Kapulanga's population was about 6,000.

It was an impoverished community, in part by virtue of the precarious economic situation of many of its residents, but also because of the lack of public services.[3] There was no school within its boundaries, no clinic or health-related out-reach programmes and no police post. Although water lines had recently been installed by the local authority, sanitation remained inadequate, with only a few scattered pit latrines. Transport was so great a problem that a resident who was sick or who had died had to be carried to the hospital. A few homes had electricity and a small number were built of concrete blocks, as were the few shops, bars, hair saloons and churches. However, most were non-permanent structures built of reeds and with mud floors. Temporary houses built of reeds were characteristic of 'traditional' modes of habitation in the province, particularly for those who routinely moved between the floodplain and its margins. However, in the context of contemporary urban life, such housing reflects relative disadvantage.

Both men and women were economically active, if often scraping to get by with meagre returns. Some of the younger members of our sample of one hundred Kapulanga residents were still financially dependent on their parents as were a few married women on their husbands. Among the rest, commerce was the predominant source of income, applying to 63 per cent of economically active women and 48 per cent of economically active men.

Commerce took a variety of forms, but women were more likely to be engaged in petty trade of fruits, vegetables and foodstuffs. Some had small stalls in Kapulanga's open air market, some sold in the market in Mongu and others from miniature stalls outside their homes. A number of women brewed opaque beer, wine, or gin, selling it to men in the numerous 'bars' which dotted the community. Men were more likely to be owners of the few shops in Kapulanga or to trade in building materials or to be involved in the outward trade in fish from the Zambezi waters and the inward trade in used clothing. Some gained income from renting houses or stalls or from artisanal activities, such as carpentry. A few cultivated plots in the vicinity of the community. A small number of both men and women were employees in Mongu, generally in low level positions. A similar number worked as traditional healers. In general, then, Kapulanga residents formed part of the informal sector of the local economic nexus, centred on Mongu but connected to the wider regional and national economy. They shifted commodities among themselves in small, sometimes minute, quantities. They engaged in wider trade networks. They provided and consumed services.

Reflecting the broader demographic profile of Mongu, almost all of those included in our baseline survey were either from ethnic groups 'indigenous' to the province and part of what Gluckman (1951) referred to as the larger Barotse nation, or from closely neighbouring areas.[4] Just over half had been born locally, with most of the others having moved from other parts of Western Province. Most (85 per cent) considered themselves to be Christian. The largest single grouping (36 per cent) was Apostolic, followed by Roman Catholics (12 per cent), but a range of other sects was also represented including the United Church of Zambia (UCZ), the Seventh Day Adventist Church (SDA) and Watchtower.

The first missionaries in the area, from the Paris Evangelical Society, remained the dominant influence for several decades. However, others subsequently entered, often establishing schools and/or hospitals, which the Lozi accepted as development goods. Shortly after Zambia's independence, in the late 1960s, there was a cluster of schools and hospitals on the eastern edge of the floodplain, in the broad vicinity of Mongu, predominantly under the auspices of the Catholic Church and UCZ (Davies, 1971). Currently, the Lewanika Hospital in Mongu, three kilometres from Kapulanga, serves as the referring hospital for the province. Among the town's secondary schools are Holy Cross and Limulunga. Mongu also has a teacher training college.

While a few households in Kapulanga were reasonably well furnished and children within them appeared to be reasonably well fed and well dressed, many children were poorly dressed and malnourished.[5] Although not specific to Kapalunga, data from Zambia's *Demographic and Health Survey 1996* (Central Statistical Office, Zambia, 1997) points to a significant deficit in children's health in the province at large. At 55.8 per 1000 births, Western Province had the highest provincial level of neonatal mortality in the country, as well as one of the highest levels of infant mortality. Perhaps most telling as an indication of poor health is that 54.7 per cent of children under five were reported to have suffered with a fever during the 2 weeks prior to the survey (considerately higher than applied in Northern Province, the 'second worst' in the country at 44.5 per cent). However, also of significance was the compromised nutritional status of women. At 19 per cent, against a national average of 9 per cent, the proportion of adult females whose body mass index was less than 18.5 kg/m was greater than in any other province.

As well as problems related to lack of transport and distance, user fees introduced in 1993 in connection with structural adjustment requirements significantly eroded access to health facilities. The number of outpatients at Lewanika Hospital dropped precipitously to 19,515 in that year from 76,220 in 1992, with a further drop in 1994 to 13,428 (Lewanika Hospital, 1994). At the same time the number of recorded cases of AIDS and AIDS-related complex at the hospital rose just as dramatically. Given cost considerations, many never approach the hospital or clinics at all. Traditional healers have been increasingly turned to for treatment of symptoms associated with HIV/ AIDS as well as other ailments, although their charges can also be prohibitive.

The picture painted by those in positions of local leadership in Kapulanga was of a community worn down by poverty and by frustration borne of an historical lack of support. Promises had been made for some years, for example, that Kapulanga should be upgraded from squatter status to become a site-and-service scheme. But delays convinced some that these promises were little more than politicians' campaigning rhetoric. The social welfare department provided small amounts of maize, sorghum and beans to a few orphans and elderly people in the community. However, apart from this, only the churches gave assistance to those who were sick, and then mainly to their own members.[6]

Local party officials and the local government councillor claimed to have personally assisted with funerals, and said they adjudicated disputes among residents. However, they lamented a general lack of community spirit and complained of limited external support. Three women's clubs set up with funds from the social welfare department, for example, were now defunct because the financial input had dried up. A neighbourhood watch group organised among youth to discourage petty thievery had waned because of lack of identity cards and withdrawal of support from the police. Whether regarding AIDS or more generally, there was little collective endeavour on the ground. When asked about groups in the area who were helping people to cope with AIDS, fifty-five of the hundred surveyed said they knew of none, four referred to anti-AIDS clubs in the schools and thirteen to churches, while twenty-five mentioned health workers or health educators.

The activities of health workers from Lewanika Hospital in Mongu were exceptionally important. They had formed a drama group to do outreach work around AIDS, after analysis of blood donated by students in local schools revealed alarmingly high levels of HIV infection, especially among girls.[7] Some of those interviewed in Kapulanga had seen and remarked on their performances. A number of other groups were also involved in AIDS work in the wider Mongu area. One was a Catholic women's organisation, Women in Society, which similarly used drama as an educational tool through plays dealing with HIV/AIDS, property-grabbing[8] and moral issues.[9] Another was, Organisation for Life, a group also associated with the Catholic church, which concentrated on facilitating AIDS awareness and behaviour change and had organised seminars in prisons, paramilitary camps, schools and at the Litunga's palace as well as youth retreats with different schools.[10] Although a branch of Organisation for Life was established in Kapulanga towards the end of the research period and several other women's and youth's groups had begun to consider adding AIDS education to their activities, for the most part members of the community neither organised themselves around AIDS nor were beneficiaries of the activities of others, save for Christian charity extended within congregations and hospital workers' educational efforts.

Indeed, the concentration of local organisations and externally supported initiatives around AIDS would appear to be less in Western Province than in other parts of Zambia. Few delegates from the province attended early national conferences of AIDS NGOs in the country. Only three of the 339 organisations, which were listed as members of the Zambia National AIDS Network in 1997 (ZNAN, 1997), were located in the province, the smallest representation of any province in the country.[11] Nor, for that matter, has much of the research conducted on HIV/AIDS in Zambia been based in or incorporated samples or case studies from Western Province.[12]

Sexuality, fertility

Cultural prescriptions regarding the specificity of gender roles, sexual behaviour and sexuality are in flux in Mongu as elsewhere, with those who are younger or have broader experience and higher levels of education being subject to a plurality of ideas about 'how to behave' and embracing a wider range of options. However, in some respects the claims of culture remain strong, given the relatively greater homogeneity of Mongu than many of Zambia's other urban areas. Change, but also greater continuity than elsewhere, can be seen in respect of initiation practices. Across Zambia as a whole, traditions of initiation of young girls and boys are becoming less important as means of providing socialisation in sexuality. That this is true of Mongu as well is suggested by data from the Kapulanga survey. Only about one-fifth of those under 20 years listed 'traditional education' as their main means for 'learning about sex', as against half of those who were older. Yet 64 per cent of males and 55 per cent of females under 20 still listed it as *one* of their sources of information on sex, suggesting that if of lesser importance, with friends of one's age competing as a primary source of information, old practices still persist in some form.

There are other ways as well in which Western Province differs from the rest of the country. For example, it has the lowest rate of fertility, save for the largely urban Lusaka Province (Central Statistical Office, Zambia, 1997). Rather than the result of delayed childbearing or more extensive use of contraception,[13] this seems to be associated with greater spacing of births, longer periods of breastfeeding, marginally longer postpartum amenorrhoea, and, especially, with longer periods of postpartum abstinence.[14]

These norms of reproductive behaviour suggest that women may be 'protected' from HIV infection for reasonably long periods after a birth.

However, such protection may be ephemeral – and certainly men's protection may be compromised – if husbands seek sexual gratification elsewhere. A strong theme emerged from focus group discussions conducted in Kapulanga that sexual intercourse was crucial to the physical and psychological well-being of both men and women. One participant, in a group of men over the age of 46,[15] said that if he were unable to have sex, he would rather be castrated, while one in a younger group of men said that without sex a person becomes 'abnormal' and, as if to emphasise its importance, said that one 'can miss meals for sex'.[16] To some degree it was accepted, even if not condoned, that men often engaged in extra-marital sexual activity, and acknowledged that (although to a much lesser extent) women were not immune from this behaviour. But it was also appreciated that, in the era of AIDS, this could be dangerous indeed.

Changing position of women

Women had strong ritual significance and formal political importance in Bulozi, as signified by the fact that for much of its history, not only was there a king resident in its main capital near Mongu, but also a princess chief presiding over its southern capital. As with the king, however, the choice of the princess chief followed the father's line and the attempt of one to install her daughter as successor was soon thwarted (Gluckman, 1951). The colonists' practice of directing attention at the Litunga under-mined the position of the princess chief (Gluckman, 1951), but her legacy and the presence of other chieftainesses within the traditional administration and the royal family provide a basis for the public respect afforded (some) women.

Gluckman's (1951, 1955) studies of the Lozi in the 1940s indicated elements of both strength and weakness in respect of the position of women. There were strong sanctions against men having physical contact with certain kinswomen. A man was considered to have committed 'adultery' if he merely walked along a path with an unrelated man's wife. Companion-ship and work relations tended to be confined within rather than across sex groupings, with men and women having little to do with each other in the public arena. A woman was legally subordinated to her husband, considered to be under his control and that of his ancestral spirits. Although women had some rights to the products of their labour, property often reverted to husbands on divorce. Yet women were held in great esteem as mothers, sisters, aunts, daughters and grand-daughters and could speak with authority. Wives were able to exert significant influence within their households. Strong ties with wives could be easily snapped, however, and often were, so that marital status was insecure.

Changes in the wider political economy gradually registered in modifica-tion of local customs, not least by virtue of extensive out-migration of men and ensuing hardship for women. In the early 1940s, it became possible for a woman to claim for divorce if her migrant husband had been away for 3 years without sending back money or goods, as against a duration of 6 years, which formerly applied (Gluckman, 1941). Over time, customs and practice continued to change. While a majority of women interviewed in Kapulanga in our 1996 survey did not own property, almost one-third of married women did, as did most of those who were divorced or widowed. Across the sample as a whole, most now consider it improper for a man to beat his wife, even if she 'misbehaved', to take her money or prevent her from working, with between three-quarters and 85 per cent routinely rejecting these propositions. Similarly, a majority felt women should be able to buy pots and pans and clothes for themselves and their children without their husband's permission. Yet the compilers of a report investigating the situation of women in Western Province, just prior to the 4th intergovernmental conference on women in Beijing in 1995, argued that many women still did not know their rights, were subject to increasing violence and faced myriad legal problems centring around marriage and property-grabbing (Republic of Zambia, Provincial Planning Unit, 1995).

The experience of AIDS: perceptions of vulnerability

How, then, has the new hazard of HIV/AIDS articulated with the pattern of continuity and change so far sketched out? How has AIDS been experienced and the danger it poses interpreted? Virtually everyone encountered in Kapulanga knew about AIDS and over two-thirds knew someone who had suffered from it, gleaning their information from such sources as: 'people discussing and seeing them suffering in the hospital'; 'seeing people suffering from it'; 'hearing many people talking about it and listening to the radio'; 'neighbours and other people talking about those sick or someone dead'; or 'seeing a friend suffer from AIDS'.[17]

Across the province as a whole, many worried that they themselves might become infected by HIV. Forty-five per cent of women (the highest provincial total in the country and contrasted with a national average of 30 per cent) believed themselves to be either at moderate or high risk of contracting HIV. The figure for men was considerably lower at 20.5 per cent but still higher than the national average for men, which was just 13 per cent (Central Statistical Office, Zambia, 1997). Of those surveyed in Kapulanga, 68 per cent of both men and women considered themselves to be in personal danger from AIDS, a strikingly high figure and indicative of the general level of anxiety, as elaborated in such comments as the following:

> I had some sexual partners years ago, so I may be infected.
> I worry whenever I have sex with a man.
> I no longer want to have sex because I fear infection.
> My husband is young; he might have extra-marital affairs and contract AIDS.

I had sex with a girl I didn't know at one of the drinking places.
Almost everyone is a victim; it is unavoidable.[18]

(Kapulanga survey respondents)

Marital status was significantly related to feelings of vulnerability[19] with 100 per cent of those who were divorced or separated, and 79 per cent of those who were married, believing themselves in danger, as against 64 per cent of those who were single and 25 per cent of those who were widowed. However, gender was also a defining factor here. Leaving aside those divorced or separated, greatest personal danger among men was perceived by those who were single, and among women, by those who were married. In total 90 per cent of married women felt themselves to be personally in danger.[20]

In considering what they might do to protect themselves, many reported that they had changed or were contemplating changing behaviour. The great majority of those surveyed confirmed that condoms were readily available in Kapulanga, but some said that they would not use them themselves and only 45 per cent agreed with the proposition that condoms offered some protection against HIV. Complaints were common in focus group discussions about condoms breaking and some believed that their 'pores' would let the virus through. However, 40 per cent of women and 53 per cent of men said that they *would* think of using condoms. While greater for those who were younger and single,[21] the proportion of married people (40 per cent) expressing willingness to use condoms was far from negligible.[22]

Yet there was evidence of a certain fatalism. In some instances, as suggested by the following comment made in a focus group discussion, the stance was almost cavalier:

Why worry or do anything? Probably all of us here are infected, but we do not know. Hence the best thing is to behave normally by fulfilling our desires. We are all at risk and those who will survive the disease are only lucky.

(Quoted in Sikwibele, 1996)

That 41 per cent of female respondents to a question about ways of avoiding AIDS in Zambia's *Demographic and Health Survey 1996* (Central Statistical Office, Zambia, 1997) said either that there was no way to avoid AIDS or that they knew of no way (as against 15 per cent of men giving this response), however, signals not just worrying gaps in knowledge, but also lack of capacity to put knowledge into practice and a sense that little is possible in any case.

Who is responsible; where does blame lie?

In Kapulanga, as elsewhere, there was a tendency for one section of the community to blame another for the spread of AIDS. Thus, married women expressed worry about contracting HIV from their husbands. But men also turned the finger of blame on women, and especially those whom they regarded as promiscuous. Rich men and young women were also frequently pointed to, as well as all those who 'moved around' and were 'careless'.

Although many believed that AIDS was brought to the province by 'strangers' or 'rich men', its subsequent transmission is largely attributed to local patterns of sexual behaviour. When asked about factors involved in the spread of AIDS, some referred to migrants returning after a period away and bringing the virus with them, a few mentioned Europeans or tourists and some said the cause was prostitution. But the major factors cited were sexual immorality (30 per cent) and 'too many partners' (45 per cent). In this regard, it was themselves, their partners, and their neighbours, who were implicated. Yet for some, particularly women and perhaps especially younger women, such improper behaviour was often contextualised in respect of poverty, so that it was not a moral defect or a matter of 'carelessness' but grounded in necessity.

The labelling, excusing and blaming, which accompany attempts to make sense of how AIDS moves through a community, can be seen in Table 3.1's summary of views of focus group participants. Vulnerability and responsibility were sometimes separated out in these accounts, but often flowed into one another. Poor women and young women were seen as both responsible for the spread of AIDS and at risk. Rich men and those having extra-marital affairs were mainly responsible, but to a lesser extent also at risk. Married women, unless they had affairs, were at risk but not necessarily responsible for the spread of AIDS. Young men could sometimes be responsible if they were reckless and 'could not control their sexual desires' but were seen as at risk if this lack of control was confined to girlfriends of their own age already infected by older, 'rich' men.

The moral ambiguity of the category 'prostitute' is also evident from these responses. Having multiple sexual encounters – five in a day or even ten in a day – and exchanging sex for livelihood are attributes which might be consistent with sex work. However, when conjoined with the element of poverty, having little choice, or pursuit by 'rich men', condemnation is muted.

The tendency for most groups to point to women as involved in and responsible for the spread of AIDS, common in many settings, is of interest for the way it contrasts with Foreman's (1999) notion of men as driving the epidemic. It is possible, however, to see this focus on women as responsible, and sometimes as blameworthy, not just in the light of their general subordination, but also in respect of a broader discourse in Lozi culture in relation to both health and the moral order. *Nyambe* (the supreme being in Lozi cosmology) was said to have placed a fixed quantity of disease in the world (Prins, 1980). While not excluding the possibility that new afflictions could enter the immediate environment, this implied an acceptance of disease as part of the natural order and not necessarily a consequence of external intrusion. Prins's (1980) account suggests that in exceptional cases, such as a smallpox epidemic of the 1890s, the nature or extent of affliction – or perhaps the

Table 3.1 Perception of responsibility and blame for AIDS from standpoints defined by gender and age[a]

Composition of group	Views of focus groups participants in Kapulanga
Female – aged 15–20	Girls of our generation because of economic insecurity and no men to marry; rich men
Female – aged 15–20	Young ladies looking for money; rich people; those coming from urban areas; uneducated people who do not know about AIDS; single ones who cannot control their sexual desires; those at risk are young unmarried women with few economic resources
Male – aged 15–20	Young girls and older men; poor women are at risk
Male – aged 15–20	Those at risk are young girls, young boys, women, town people and unmarried people; poverty is the cause in the case of women
Female – aged 21–45	Men are responsible; but poverty makes women 'reckless'
Female – aged 21–45	Women needing money; but both males and females; businessmen who travel, youths; educated people; town dwellers; women with no income are at risk
Male – aged 21–45	Women 'following any man' and asking for sexual favours for their livelihood; young girls going for rich men; rich men with money to dish out
Female – aged 46+	Women who don't say no to men and exchange sex for money; older men and younger girls; married women are at risk
Male – aged 46+	Elderly men and women having sex with young girls and boys; rich people; educated and town dwellers; married women having extra-marital affairs; women who have sex up to five times a day
Mixed	Both men and women, especially women having sex ten times a day for survival; both old and young; rich men; educated; town people

[a] *Source*: focus group discussions, Kapulanga, 1996.

elusiveness of successful treatment – placed it beyond the norm, requiring a communal response involving functions at the royal graves. More generally, however, individuals endeavoured to avoid disease by observing taboos.

What concerns us here is that taboos relating to women's reproductive system – and especially menstruation or post-parturition – were particularly important in explaining certain afflictions. While differing in specifics, this resonates with the beliefs of other groups in the region. When sexual relations took place with a woman who had not been ritually cleansed[23] (and was therefore considered unclean) after an abnormal event such as an abortion, miscarriage or stillbirth, or when taboos regarding sexual abstinence at prescribed times were breached, illness or affliction could result. Men were implicated in breaking taboos through having sexual relations with a women at improper times, and in the process could themselves become afflicted. However, the state of danger was specifically defined in terms of women's condition. The 'cause' was located with women, with men being 'victims'. Embedded ideas about the dangers of sexual behaviour breaching conventional norms, and the connection drawn between illness and women's physiology, may have thus predisposed women to be blamed in respect of a new and deadly illness involving transmission via sexual intercourse.

Among the Lozi (and again elsewhere) entrenched attitudes which placed primary responsibility for marital infidelity on women further encouraged such a response. In his analysis of the Lozi judicial system in the 1940s, Gluckman (1955) describes how Lozi men, including male jurists, blamed women, whose behaviour they contrasted unfavourably with the moral uprightness of their own 'mothers', for what they believed to be a worrying increase in premarital pregnancies, adultery and divorce. Moreover, they typically regarded prostitution as a vice of women, associated with and reflecting women's licentiousness and avarice. While Gluckman confirms that these were contested views, the power exerted by male jurists in upholding their prejudices necessarily contributed to a general legal subjection of wives in Lozi society.

The process of social change captured by Gluckman in the 1940s has continued to unfold, but a degree of continuity can be detected in the way in which judgements about blame are fundamentally shaped by gendered power relations within society. While there may be increasing admission that all are implicated and greater appreciation of the social and economic factors which put some individuals into positions of vulnerability, certain prejudices remain.

Difference in perception according to standpoint

It is of interest in this regard that while qualifying their remarks with a reference to poverty and to the power relations exerted by husbands or rich men, or indeed men in general, women so frequently indicted their own gender as responsible for the spread of AIDS. In practice this reflects divisions among women and antagonism of (some) older women towards those younger women judged as showing insufficient respect for 'traditional morality'. It also reflects the antagonism of (some) married women to sex workers or to any who are 'reckless' and exchange sex, even if for material gain, outside of marriage. But some married women conceded that these divisions could be permeable and that, if not themselves as individuals, then their fellow married women should also shoulder some personal responsibility for the spread of AIDS. Women should be strong. Hence the view of those in the focus group of older women (aged 46 years and above):

> Women are responsible for the spread of AIDS. They are the ones with the power to say no to men, but they are more interested in getting money from men and therefore engage in prostitution and careless sex with tourists.
>
> (Kapulanga focus group)[24]

For their part young women seemed almost to accept their powerlessness in the situation in which they found themselves. It is striking how willing they were to admit the complicity of their generation in the spread of AIDS and, at the same time, how convinced they were of the links between responsibility, vulnerability and economic dependence. The unanimous conclusion of one group, was that 'improved economic status for both girls and women will help protect them as they would have their own means of livelihood and rely less on men'.[25]

Men acknowledged their own involvement with activities which facilitated the spread of AIDS. Yet some continued both to excuse this as part of their nature and to blame the women with whom they had sex. While manoeuvring themselves into a place of lesser blame, they could also harbour a sense of awe at women's sexual endurance, all the while conceding that such women's behaviour was not based on greed or lack of sexual control, but economic need. Thus, as one commented:

> Both men and women are responsible for the spread of AIDS, but especially women who can manage to have sex with ten men in a day in order to have money for their survival.[26]

Young men were least likely to regard themselves or be regarded as primarily responsible for the spread of AIDS. Indeed in some respects they were perceived as victims of the unguarded activities of rich or older men who seduced younger women with the promise of material gain. Some of these young men, both as survey respondents or focus group participants, were clearly traumatised by the threat of AIDS and referred to the fear that they might be infected through sex with their girlfriends: 'maybe my girlfriend might bring it to me although I try to behave well'.[27] However, they seemed to focus on self protection and the possibility of accidental infection, rather than exhibit concern that their pursuit of pleasure might lead to the further transmission of HIV. While some said that they would use a condom 'whenever I want to have sex'; or 'all the time as long as I am not married'; or 'when I will be sexually active',[28] others commented that they would only use them 'when I suspect the girlfriend' or 'when I know and suspect that my partner has other sexual partners'.[29] And two, who earlier in the interview admitted that they had had previous sexual encounters and might therefore be already infected, said that they would not use condoms.[30]

This image of young men as more likely to be unwitting victims than primary transmitters of HIV contrasts with Setel's (1996) account of responses to AIDS in Kilimanjaro in Tanzania. In that case the behaviour of young men was seen as implicated in a loosening of the moral fabric and basic integrity of the community, which presaged the entry of AIDS. In Kapulanga, the sexual behaviour of young men was broadly left uncontested, unless so extensive as to warrant the judgement that they were 'not in control' of their sexual urges. There are limits to how far this contrast can be taken. However, it may provide a glimpse of the way that AIDS insinuates itself into different social contexts in different ways and with different outcomes, highlighting points of social tension and exposing the gender dynamics of social and economic change.

Concluding comments

This account of Kapulanga's experience of AIDS has emphasised a high level of need, given indicators showing Western Province generally to have poorer health than other parts of Zambia and Mongu, in particular, to have disturbingly high HIV prevalence. In looking at the historical and cultural context, we have attempted to show how the retention by traditional authorities of an unusual degree of cultural and political autonomy set the scene for tension between province and national government which continues to the present. Repeated complaints of central government's neglect of the area appear to have contemporary parallel in a dearth of local interventions around AIDS. Toward the end of the research period there was a flurry of activity in Kapulanga, with acceptance of a proposal from the local health advisory committee that a clinic should be established there and residents involved in making bricks for more permanent structures. On the back of such activity, optimism was generated that collective action around AIDS might also be set in motion.[31]

Perhaps it was more than coincidental, however, that these positive signs occurred in the midst of the campaign for national presidential and parliamentary elections, which saw a range of overtures from the ruling party to residents of a province where there were strong signs of local political opposition. In the event, a decidedly mixed electoral result in Western Province, with as many seats going to opposition parties or independent candidates as to the ruling party, may have cooled the relationship between province and central government, with the subsequent renewal of calls by traditionalists for reinstatement of the old Barotseland Agreement reflecting persistent unease. National policies to devolve government AIDS programmes to the locality might hold some promise for communities such as Kapulanga, but only if local infrastructure is introduced and support extended to match local initiative.

Our account has also attempted to examine responses to AIDS in terms of embedded cultural practices and beliefs connecting illness with taboos associated with women's reproductive physiology and 'improper' sexual behaviour. We have noted that, even if in decline, there is greater retention of 'traditional' sexual initiation in Western Province than in many other parts of the country, indicating the continuing salience and integrity of a strong cultural tradition. A tendency to view women as disproportionately responsible for moral decline has contributed to contemporary patterns of blame and recrimination in the context of AIDS. And yet, while all bear responsibility, it is women who remain predominantly at risk.

Notes

1 Kapulanga survey 1996.
2 Research upon which this chapter is written was carried out between July 1995 and November 1996 by Caroline Shonga and Anne Sikwibele. They were assisted by Mrs Wakalala (in September 1995), Elizabeth Mukwita and Miriam Mundia (in early 1996 in carrying out the baseline survey), M. Sifuniso and Kapenda Kapenda (in April 1996 in facilitating focus group discussions) and G. Mweene and Kanjumbo Yikwayabo (in late 1996 in facilitating group work around AIDS in Kapulanga). A number of interviews were carried out in conjunction with the research, with school teachers, health workers, chemists, traditional healers, officers in the provincial government, local councillors, women's groups, church officials, and community leaders in Kapulanga. In accord with the overall protocol for the research, a baseline survey was conducted early in 1996, with one hundred respondents chosen according to specified criteria (see Chapter 2). Ten focus groups were carried out with men and women of the same age categories which define the baseline sample (15–19, 21–45 and 46+).
3 This section is based on interviews with a range of community leaders carried out in July 1995 and January 1996.
4 Thirty-five per cent specifically identified themselves as Lozi and a further 12 per cent, as either Kwandi or Kwangwa. Twenty per cent were Mbunda and 5 per cent Nkoya. Finally, 15 per cent were Lubale from north of the province.
5 Field notes, research team.
6 This at least was the consensus view of a number of informants (interviews January 1996).
7 Research diary and interview, C. Shonga, 19 July 1995.
8 Property grabbing refers to the custom, now illegal in respect of civil marriages in Zambia, of a husband's relatives claiming and removing his property on his death, in some cases even property which has been jointly owned.
9 Research diary, C. Shonga, July 1995.
10 Interview, 24 October 1996; interview with members, 25 October 1996.
11 The Network's membership, which included government departments and some international organisations among its members, as well as NGOs, does not constitute a comprehensive list of AIDS activities and it is probable that local initiatives in provinces away from Zambia's line-of-rail are inhibited from joining by virtue of problems of communication and, indeed, distance. Yet the meagre listing for Western Province is indicative of a lower level of activity, which matches the findings of the research team.

12 In the geographical index of Zambia's HIV/AIDS Bibliography (NASTLP and UNICEF, 1996), only western and north-western Provinces have no listings.
13 Only 2 per cent of married women reported using condoms as a contraceptives, the second lowest provincial average in the country. Only 19 per cent reported using 'any method' of contraception (Central Statistical Office, Zambia, 1997).
14 The median figure across the province for postpartum abstinence was 13.1 months as against a national average of 8.3 months (Central Statistical Office, Zambia, 1997).
15 Kapulanga focus group, men 46 and above, 29 April 1996, facilitator, M. Sifuniso.
16 Kapulanga focus group, men 20–45, 28 April 1996, facilitator, M. Sifuniso.
17 Kapulanga survey respondents.
18 Kapulanga survey 1996.
19 The chi-square statistic for marital status and personal danger was significant at 17.6, d.f. $= 3$, $p = 0.00$.
20 While not significant for men, there was a significant relationship for women between marital status and sense of personal danger, but numbers are too small for this result to taken as reliable.
21 The chi-square statistic for age and willingness to use condoms was significant but numbers are too small for this result to be taken as reliable.
22 However, the relationship was not significant for marital status and willingness to use condoms.
23 Cleansing may take various forms according to conventions.
24 Women 46 and above, 19 April 1996, facilitator, A. Sikwibele.
25 Kapulanga, focus group, women 15–19, 30 April 1996, facilitator, A. Sikwibele.
26 Kapulanga, focus group, mixed group, 3 May 1996, facilitator, Mr Kapenda.
27 Kapulanga survey respondent.
28 Kapulanga survey respondents.
29 Kapulanga survey respondents.
30 Kapulanga survey respondents.
31 Field notes, November 1996.

4 Sinners and outsiders: the drama of AIDS in Rungwe

Marjorie Mbilinyi and Naomi Kaihula[1]

Local communities in Rungwe district, Mbeya, are grappling with the effects of HIV/AIDS during a time of major crisis in the smallholder farm economy and marked shifts in the balance of economic power between men and women. The HIV/AIDS epidemic has spread throughout Rungwe. It is prevalent in peri-urban trade centres along the main highway linking Malawi to Tanzania, which cuts right across the district. It is also found in villages scattered along the numerous 'tea roads' built to facilitate the flow of green leaf tea from smallholder farms to the Katumba tea factory. Mbeya region ranks highest in Tanzania in terms of officially reported accumulated AIDS cases (NACP, 1998b: 11).

In the 1970s, Rungwe had a flourishing rural economy based on smallholder coffee and tea, waged employment in the Tukuyu tea estates and the Kiwira coal mine, along with wage remittances from migrant workers. Smallholder coffee and tea have collapsed as a result of structural adjustment policies, and jobs in the government and parastatal sector have been lost in consequence of retrenchment and privatisation. Privileged in the past because of their control over tea and coffee crops and greater access to wage employment, men have experienced a radical decline in income, whereas women have become increasingly involved in cash earning activities.

One of the main arguments of this chapter is that women have become more economically autonomous during recent years, and youth (both male and female) have rebelled against the control of their elders. This has had repercussions for sexual behaviour and subsequently for HIV/AIDS. The balance of power at household level is shifting, albeit slowly and unevenly, as a growing number of rural households have come to depend on women's incomes for daily subsistence needs (Kaihula, 1995; Mbilinyi, 1997). Changing gender relations construct responses to HIV/AIDS as AIDS reconstructs gender relations.

Our second main argument is that religion, namely Protestant Christianity, has framed the discourses within which morality and sexuality are debated and acted out in Rungwe, with often contradictory responses to the epidemic. Strong religious principles and doctrine govern people's overt moral, sexual and cultural behaviour (Kalindile and Mbilinyi, 1991). Prohibitions against

alcohol consumption and extramarital sexual relations take special precedence, along with positive promotion of community support for the sick
and dying. The church upholds male dominance within marriage, while at
the same time providing women with some opportunity to assert themselves
as leaders within the church hierarchy.

As young and old, women and men, try to make sense of the AIDS disaster
through developing coping strategies (Barnett and Blaikie, 1992), they draw
on already existing knowledge and belief systems in Christianity and local
Nyakyusa culture. In Rungwe, as elsewhere, one way that people cope is to
blame others, and to look for ways of excluding them. They may eject them
from the family or the community, deny them adequate support and assistance, or exclude them psychologically through stigmatisation or discrimination. These forms of exclusion correspond to the concept of abjection
developed by Kristeva (1982) and applied by Zivi (1998) to the AIDS
phenomenon. The abject is that object or person that is perceived to be a
threat to social order, and is often associated with filth, waste, bodily fluids or
death. A community/society adopts mechanisms to separate and divide so as
to expel the abject, which is referred to as abjection.

The boundaries which define who is immoral and who is pure are
constructed with reference to existing abjected groups, i.e. marginalised categories. In Rungwe this means sex workers, outsiders, unruly young men,
women traders and certain kinds of 'other' women. These responses undermine efforts to protect the human rights of people with HIV/AIDS and their
families, and to develop more effective coping strategies for prevention and
care. At the same time, the abjection process in Rungwe is counteracted by
Christian principles of compassion for the sick and the poor, and ideal images
of female nurturance towards husbands, children and other members of the
household and community.

An historical approach has been adopted to help situate and explain the
construction of the present AIDS crisis. The Nyakyusa people of Rungwe
have experienced several ruptures in their history, including military conquest
by the Germans, economic restructuring and the addition of Christian philo-
sophy to a strong Nyakyusa belief system based on ancestor worship. Local
interpretations and responses to AIDS are partly determined by earlier struggles shaped by these developments, and often centre on the control of women
and youth.

Study location and research activities

Field work was carried out from July 1995 to February 1996 in three wards of
Rungwe district: Katumba, Kiwira and Kisondela. In Katumba, the greatest
focus was on Katumba village, situated about 10 km from the district headquarters, Tukuyu, and along the paved highway between Mbeya and the
Malawi border, a regular stop for bus travellers and lorry drivers. The
presence of the Katumba tea factory and the highway has altered the social

landscape, making it more cosmopolitan, with a mix of ethnic groups. Now a significant trading centre, Katumba has three guest houses, several modern bars and home brew beer huts, shops, a daily market and a variety of street stalls where traders sell everything from soap, pens and condoms to fresh fruits and vegetables.

Few full-time farmers are left in the village community surrounding the factory. Women and men have become increasingly involved in off-farm activities. Most local shops are owned by Nyakyusa men, whereas Nyakyusa women are involved in trade, beer brewing, food preparation and sale. The factory has attracted newcomers seeking income as employees, but also as sex workers and traders. They come from other villages in the district as well as from non-Nyakyusa ethnic groups, the Ngoni, Chagga and Haya.

Several other villages in Katumba Ward were also included in the research. Most important amongst these were Iringa, about 4 km off the main highway and Ikama, about 3 km from the road running from the Katumba factory to Mwakaleli. The majority in both were smallholders, although a few were casual workers on the Tukuyu tea estates and at the Katumba factory. Women also traded at weekly markets, which drew crop buyers and traders from as far afield as Mbeya and Dar es Salaam.

Kiwira Ward lies along the Mbeya-Tukuyu highway, not far from Katumba. Its development has been influenced by the Kiwira coal mine and trade centres which emerged nearby. It is also the site of Rungwe mission, the centre of the entire Moravian church in the district. Villages focused on here were Mpandapanda, Syukula, Kyimo and Kiwira. Finally, Kisondela Ward, where we visited Kisondela village, is another major centre for the Moravian church.

A variety of research methods were used, as described in Chapter 2. Of greatest importance were focus group discussions where different social groups shared information, perceptions and feelings about HIV/AIDS, its causes and its prevention. Several were impromptu, such as one involving thirteen men at a funeral in Ikama and others with sex workers, divorced women, male and female Lutengano secondary school students, and female and male bar attendants. Others were arranged more formally, often with the active support of institutional leaders. These included discussions with ward officers at Katumba, Lugambo and Kidondela; district community development officers; HIV/AIDS health workers, counsellors and educators at Makandana Hospital in Tukuyu; and workers at Igogwe and Itete AIDS counselling centres. Staff attached to religious institutions were also interviewed: at the Lutheran headquarters in Tukuyu; the Moravian seminary at Lutengano in Kisondela Ward; and the Rungwe Moravian headquarters in Kiwira Ward. Finally, meetings were held with church groups, such as the Lutheran Women's Group and the Galilaya Assemblies of God youth and women's group in Katumba.

In 1995, a total of fifty men and fifty women were interviewed using the stratified sampling frame and structured interview schedule described in

Chapter 2. Finally, awareness-raising and feedback seminars were organised by Kaihula and her assistant, Mwaipopo, in 1995 and 1996 at a variety of locations, often with large numbers of participants. These ranged from forty-five people at Katumba primary school to two hundred and ninety at Tukuyu Teachers College; and from sixteen members of Galilaya Women's Group to eighty-two men and women at Katumba Primary Court. The seminars were organised in a lively fashion, with formal presentations, demonstrations of condom use, group discussions, and formal presentations not only by the two researchers, but by local AIDS counsellors. Much of the seminar time was devoted to an exchange of views about AIDS, how people protect themselves, and problems pertaining to sexuality. Nearly all seminars included both women and men, providing a unique opportunity to discuss issues of sexual behaviour and relationships together. A total of five hundred and twenty-four and four hundred and twenty people participated in seminars during 1995 and 1996, respectively, of whom 56 per cent were women.

The changing context of Rungwe

What troubled many participants in the study was the fast pace of social change, which they perceived to be beyond their control. Rungwe has indeed experienced economic crisis and attendant changes in the gender division of labour during the last 20 years, following an earlier history of social and economic transformations associated with colonisation and the post-colonial process of 'development'.

Rungwe flourished between the sixteenth and nineteenth centuries, protected from the worst vagaries of the slave trade. Fertile soil, ample rainfall and many springs and rivers contributed to a thriving banana-based economy, with a large variety of basic food crops. A strong patrilineal and patrilocal system developed, with a combination of chiefly and clan rule. Princes ruled in conjunction with commoner elders, the *mafumu*, and had major judiciary powers with respect to what are today distinguished as criminal and civil misdemeanours (Wilson, 1955). Sexual behaviour was governed through patriliny, polygamy, bridewealth, child brides, and widow inheritance (Katapa, 1998).

Women and men had complementary responsibilities for production of basic food stuffs. Men were responsible for heavy clearing, wood-cutting and cultivation; women carried out planting, weeding and harvesting. Men also herded and milked cattle. Women carried water from the many rivers, streams and springs, and firewood from nearby forests.

The inroads of European colonisation altered this situation. German military conquest in the late 1880s was accompanied by missionary activity of the Moravian and Lutheran churches. Economic pressures became the major source of change – a combination of forced taxation of adult males, coercive cultivation of certain crops and appropriation of land by white settler farmers to grow coffee and later tea. Under British rule, a migrant labour system was organised to provide cheap African labour to the then Rhodesian Copperbelt and the Johannesburg gold mines (Mbilinyi, 1991). At any one moment during the 1940s and 1950s, at least a quarter of 'young' adult males were absent on the mines.

The gender division of labour began to change during this time. With the departure of men as migrant labourers, women were forced to carry out former male functions such as land clearing, the cutting of fuel logs and even the construction of houses. Responsibility for maintaining and assisting the households of migrant workers was left in the hands of in-laws. This left 'grass widows' under surveillance, their sexual behaviour monitored and controlled. At the wider community level, the power and revenue of the princes – now called chiefs – became increasingly dependent on their judicial role in the regulation of marriage, divorce, inheritance and allocation of land within the tribe's territory. The politics of reproduction and sexuality were therefore heightened.

Another division developed, between cash crops for export (coffee), controlled by men, and food crops, which were redefined as women's responsibility. Smallholder production of coffee spread among local inhabitants, under the control of male household heads but fully dependent on the unpaid labour of wives, children and other dependants. Women maintained the banana groves and were allocated their own fields to grow family food, sweet potatoes, cocoyams and beans.

Many men and women became Christian converts, forcing a major break with Nyakyusa customs and beliefs (Kalindile and Mbilinyi, 1991). The Moravian church's institutional structure was semi-democratic: both women and men were chosen to become church elders, and representatives of local village churches were chosen to sit in the top synod. At the same time, men dominated church hierarchies, and an extremely patriarchal interpretation of the Bible was in force then, as now. Race divisions were also marked. European missionaries dominated the preaching and overall administration, relegating local Africans to catechist positions for many years.

Marriage systems and sexual practices were affected by religious conversion and wider economic changes. From the 1930s to the 1950s, the practice of widow inheritance declined, particularly within Christian communities. Although girls continued to be betrothed as infants or young girls, they did not move to the homes of their husbands until they reached puberty (Katapa, 1998). Divorce became more common, as women began to move more freely between town and country as traders, and followed husbands or lovers to the mines.

Immediately after independence in 1961, men lost a major source of employment and income as a result of a government ban on southward labour migration. At the same time, restrictions against Africans growing tea were lifted, and with World Bank support, smallholder tea production became a key cash earner in Rungwe, under the control of male household heads.

Katumba tea factory was built at this time by the Tanzania Tea Authority, which controlled the marketing of smallholder tea. A dense network of 'tea roads' was constructed throughout Rungwe district, which also enhanced the movement of women banana traders and later facilitated the development of weekly markets. Private company-owned tea estates continued to operate in the area, but faced severe labour shortages arising from the expansion of smallholder tea production.

Socialist policies and villagisation strategies from 1967 onwards represented another external interference in the local community. Although forced resettlement was not attempted in any of the densely populated highlands areas, including Rungwe, the political and economic landscape changed, with growing power in the hands of local leaders of the ruling party and local government authorities. Villagers were now expected to work on village collective farms and other projects, as well as to participate in block farming (where proceeds remained in their own hands). Whereas communal labour was once mobilised by the colonial chiefs, it was now organised by village leaders, although there was some overlap in personnel between 'traditional' and contemporary state structures.

Women were enthusiastic about some aspects of villagisation. Block farming of tea, for example, gave them direct control over the cash proceeds of their cultivation, whilst the ousting of private traders and village control over maize surplus sales ensured access to food at reasonable prices during 'bad times' (Mbilinyi, 1991). Village and women's co-operative shops replaced private shopkeepers, and during the period of severe shortages of goods (late 1970s to early 1980s) were often the sole source of basic commodities such as kerosene, *khanga* cloth and sugar. Parallel marketing and smuggling of goods back and forth over the Malawian and Zambian borders also flourished, and local women became major actors in long distance trade (ibid.; Katapa, 1998). Access to basic social services also expanded. Rural health clinics were established in every ward, and universal primary education opened the doors to formal education for the first time to most Nyakyusa girls. These services were provided free in the case of health, and at a very low cost in the case of education.

Structural adjustment and liberalisation policies were adopted by the government in the mid 1980s after a seven year struggle with donors, led by the World Bank and IMF. According to local perceptions, SAPs had some positive consequences: the flooding of local markets with imported second-hand clothes, the removal of barriers to local entrepreneurship and micro-small enterprises, and later, the liberalisation of tea and coffee marketing. Conversely, producer prices for tea and coffee declined and smallholder growers no longer had access to a regular supply of credit in cash and kind to secure tea seedlings and fertiliser. Poverty and income inequalities deepened. Most poignant of all, the gains made in universal primary education were lost, as a result of cost sharing policies. Public provision of health services was eroded, with charges putting them beyond the means of poor households.

Smallholder farming could no longer absorb the labour of most grown children, and declining returns made farming less attractive to the young. This led to a rapid rise in un-/underemployment particularly among male youth, the increased involvement of young men in petty business and theft, and women of all ages in off-farm activities such as beer brewing, prostitution and trade. In the next section, we examine the phenomenon of women's economic empowerment in more detail.

Women's economic empowerment? A new trend in Rungwe

Many women in our study, whether married or unmarried, earned independent cash incomes on the basis of beer brewing/sale, and trade in bananas, second-hand clothes and other goods.[2] Not only did a growing number of women engage in independent micro-small enterprises, but a few had become relatively wealthy entrepreneurs (Kaihula, 1995). Nyakyusa business women owned shops, tea houses, restaurants, hotels, salons, tailoring businesses, transport companies and dairy farms, mainly in Tukuyu, Mbeya town and urbanised trade centres. Few well-to-do business women remained locked in oppressive marriage relationships. Many rejected marriage, or else insisted on more equitable relations. Given the decline of male incomes in agriculture and the loss of well-paid positions in the formal labour market, some men had adapted and become supportive help-mates.

In the villages visited, many women controlled their own cash, and some husbands had to beg or borrow. If a man wanted his wife to wash his clothes, he had to provide the soap. Elderly wives said that they did not request permission to do things or go places; rather, they 'informed' their husbands as a matter of 'courtesy' and mutual respect. Another indicator of women's new power was their capacity to build their own houses and to educate their children. Some had provided modern roofing material for parents, and even built separate houses for husbands.

Some women, both married and unmarried, had turned to sex work. An index of the poverty of many, it also provided the means to prosper for the few. Poor married, divorced and widowed women looked to exchange sex for food as well as money. Rather than abjectify women as sinners for engaging in sex work, many people viewed the conditions which forced women to take such steps, as beyond their control. They were the consequence of drunken husbands who neglected their wife(ves) and spent whatever money they had on alcohol and commercial sex, or of in-laws who deprived widows of their land and homes, and sometimes their children. Local patrilineal systems denied women independent access to land from their families of origin. Divorced or dispossessed, they returned as dependants of elderly parents, and were subjugated to brothers, younger or older. As one woman said:

'they are better off beer brewing and living off boyfriends, than going back home to be brutally treated by their brothers!'.

Some women used the savings from sex work and the beer trade as capital to build houses or expand business. Men and women referred to the boom period of 1992–93 when 'foreign' workers from outside the area came to construct the highway. Women beer brewers/sex workers converged on the construction camps that were established in Kiwira and Ilima. Three women friends living in Iringa village used their proceeds from beer sales at this period to jointly purchase a pick-up and establish a business selling bananas in Zambia and Kilombero. They returned with fish and sugar from Kilombero and soap from Zambia to sell in local markets. Many of these women were divorced or widowed household heads, but others were married.

Struggles to control women and male youth

Elders frequently spoke of their loss of control over the sexual behaviour of youth and women, linking this to a general breakdown of social order and the generational hierarchy. Male elders complained that the younger generation could not be supervised, taught or assisted because 'they did not listen to their elders'; 'youth have totally changed'. One man pointed to the loss of traditional knowledge about alternative sexual practices: 'There is no need to stress condom use for youth. If they only listened to and respected the teaching of the elders, we could tell them other ways of getting sexual release without penetrating a woman'.

Loss of control over young people's labour power was also emphasised. During the focus group discussion in Iringa, women elders spoke of how: 'young people do not want to work on the farm, all they want to do is go watch videos'; 'they want to get things free'; 'when we old people pass away, there will be no more farmers because the young people do not want to farm'. In reply, one young man highlighted the problems of trying to carry out independent income-earning activities within the orbit of the household economy: 'if one starts a project like a market garden, he will be forced to bow to his parents. His mother will start harvesting the vegetables for herself or the family, and he will suffer a loss'. Another complained that they were used as unpaid labour force on their parents' farms. 'When we help, they discourage us by not paying us anything. We say to our fathers, "you sell the coffee, why don't you share some of the proceeds? You only buy soap for yourself and your wife". We explain to our mothers, "you sell the bananas, but no soap for us'. Another young man asked why they could not be allocated a plot from the family farm while their fathers were still alive. In response older women bemoaned the tendency of young men to depend on their mothers for food, without contributing to 'the pot' in cash or kind or labour – a contrasting example of exploitation of unpaid family labour. Young people increasingly seek off-farm sources of income beyond the grasp of their parents (Mbilinyi, 1991, 1997), their behaviour beyond parental control. A growing number of young women refuse to marry, saying that they would not agree to be men's slaves. By contrast, young men claimed that they could not afford to marry, as they could not compete with relatively better-off older men in provision of bridewealth, land and other assets. Girls who sought the supposed stability and security of marriage might therefore become second or third wives to older men, compounding their risk of being infected by HIV/AIDS (Mbilinyi, 1991).

Most alarming to men appeared to be a loss of control over wives, especially traders who travelled to distant urban centres to sell bananas and purchase other commodities, such as second-hand clothes, for sale in the village markets. 'These women traders go out of husbands' and relatives' control – it is easy to conduct love affairs'. They pointed out that many of the places where women traded were areas with high levels of seroprevalence, including Zambia, Malawi, Kyela, Mbeya town and Chunya district. It was alleged that most people who died of AIDS in the village were single women who had been trading outside of Rungwe. The same was said of seropositive men, however – they had gone to live and trade elsewhere, or to mine in Zambia or Chunya, or to work in the sugar-cane plantations of Kilombero. Here the dangers of going outside are emphasised, with respect to both women and men – outside the local community, outside the control of male elders. This has been noted also in Lushoto (Bujra, 2000a).

Men reacted to these changes in gender relations with resentment and fear. Husbands were now pressed to take on female responsibilities, such as child rearing, bathing children, and cultivating food for the household. They had to devise cover stories: 'Oh my wife is away, she's working in Mbeya'. Local women traders also allegedly bought the sexual services of young men, thus further upsetting the 'normal' sexual hierarchy. The normal had become abnormal in gender and sexual relations, as many men, especially those in poor economic conditions, found themselves increasingly dependent on the income earnings of their wives, sisters, mothers, daughters.

Laments of old men over the loss of control over youth and women are not new. Colonial archives and oral histories document major concern about loss of control, beginning especially in the 1930s and 1940s, with the expansion of the migrant labour system (Mbilinyi, 1991). Elders and chiefs lost control over the labour of male youth, who could earn independent incomes in the mines and purchase cattle for bridewealth, thus sidestepping elder domination and control over property, bridewealth and wives. Perceptions of HIV/AIDS and its causes reflected the same concern over a world turned upside down, with women and youth apparently free to do as they wish, without regard to their own safety, let alone that of their partners.

Satan and the loss of tradition

Christian and indigenous polarities of good and evil, holiness and sin, framed the dominant discourse through which HIV/AIDS was constructed in

Rungwe. More than half of the participants in the study belonged to the local Moravian church, which structures the life of the entire community. Discussions around causality aroused a series of responses expressing the idea of abjection. Everyone associated AIDS with their own version of high-risk groups: youth (male and female), sex workers, women traders and barmaids, and outsiders (factory workers, truck drivers). The drivers of the big container trucks were especially feared by local people as bearers of infection.

Risky sexual practices were also highlighted: promiscuity among youth (mentioned by older women and men); and men (as noted by women); multiple sex partners among husbands (as reported by married women); and widow inheritance. Risky places included local beer clubs, weekly or shifting markets, local dances, and the highway, which loomed large as the route by which outsiders entered and the means by which women went outside.

Monetisation and the breakdown of 'tradition'

A common theme in discussions was the link between perceived sexual laxity, the breakdown of 'traditional' systems, and money (a discourse also noted in Uganda by Weiss, 1993). Male elders deplored the impact of the money economy on traditional social relations. 'Society has lost cohesion, money has caused the erosion of traditions'. 'Today the community lacks the unity to deal with lazy people, drunks and prostitutes#'. One elderly woman said that, 'Children of today do not listen because they are fond of money. Moreover, there is no longer any kind of sexual education for young girls, whether married or unmarried'. The elders remarked that in the past, girls did not engage in sexual relationships before marriage, whereas these days, there was no controlling them.

However, both positive and negative views of 'tradition' were expressed, especially by women. They criticised traditional practices such as the acceptance of male promiscuity. And one traditional custom, polygamy, was considered by many women to be dangerous under present circumstances. Since the husband could only serve one wife at a time, polygamy did not provide co-wives with adequate sexual pleasure, leaving the others neglected and tempted to seek alternative lovers. On the other hand, young women might accept polygamous marriage in order to acquire economic status, whilst earlier sexual partnerships with young lovers were sustained, thus endangering the lives of everyone in the marriage.

Men, on the other hand, accused women of breaking with the past and thereby bringing and sustaining HIV/AIDS. Traditional patterns of marriage were no longer followed. Women 'even ran with foreigners [road construction workers and truck drivers]'. 'The girls are the worst, they do not want to marry the Nyakyusas, they want foreigners only. Some bring husbands from man-eating tribes'. 'The girls are hungry for money, and have no desire to follow the old traditions'.

When young women respond they often sound angry and defensive. In a focus group in Katumba village, one young woman said that girls were seduced by old men with the promise of material things. She insisted that since everyone was a hooligan or prostitute (*mhuni*), no-one was in a position to point a finger at anyone else. Similar accusations were made against elderly male sugar daddies by young women in Kiwira, Kipoke village and Lutengano secondary school.

Women banana traders in Kiwira also rejected being scapegoated as HIV carriers, claiming that they received education and were getting medical check-ups on a regular basis.[3] In group discussions everywhere, women and men both agreed that it was not fair to single out women traders. Young men also went outside to hunt for gold in Chunya and Songea, or to seek wage employment in Zambia and South Africa or on the plantations in Kilombero and Mtera, and brought HIV back with them. The theme of outsiders/those who go outside as abject is linked to money, the breaking of traditional order, modernisation, and ultimately, the autonomy – however contradictory – of (young) women. Where the emphasis fell depended on the gender/age of the speaker. The choice of words and symbols was expressive of conflicts and tensions at many levels: women run with foreigners; men from man-eating tribes; girls hungry for money-eating, hunger, sex. In particular the AIDS issue is used as an opportunity by some to critique Rungwe women's expanded economic power.

AIDS as sin

In Rungwe, AIDS discourse is also permeated by Christian views of morality, especially amongst adherents of the more fundamentalist sects. Religious songs of the Galilaya Youth (Assemblies of God) condemn, 'the evil of AIDS' as the product of an 'adulterous life'. Youthful members of their congregations often take the lead in these denunciations, as if to distance themselves from generally negative views of youth. Church members and leaders in Rungwe not only blamed the youth and unfaithful for their sinning ways, but also parents for being lax in moral education of their children. Mothers, especially, were said to be preoccupied with economic endeavours.

These views resonate with those expressed by Christian leaders elsewhere in the country. At a Bishops' conference in 1987, AIDS was characterised as God's punishment for the sins of human beings. A Christian pastor blamed youth's 'moral laxity' for the spread of AIDS, and their attraction to video shows, music, loose dressing and urban life in general (Christian Council of Tanzania, 1987). Christian leaders use Biblical quotations to support their arguments, such as Deuteronomy 25, which carries prophecies of the plagues and calamities to befall sinners who break God's law.

A bitter, mean-spirited and punitive ideology has thus been constructed by some church leaders and lay persons to cope with AIDS. By linking AIDS with transgression, it abjects from decent human society the rebellious young, the modernised and those resistant to church (and elderly) authority. These views resonate with Watney's (1988: 80) discussion of AIDS as spectacle or pageant, 'a purgative ritual in which we see the evildoers punished, while the national family unit – understood as the locus of the 'the social' – is cleansed and restored'. Whilst highlighting the divide between mainstream heterosexual hegemony vis-a-vis homosexuality, Watney's analysis is also relevant to the abjection process taking place in Tanzanian communities and national institutions – though here, the values and aspirations of young people for all things modern and 'global' are part of a mainstream discourse, not that of a marginalised minority.

Conflict and compassion in the churches

The moral crusade against AIDS was by no means greeted with unanimity. Divisions within churches, between elders/leaders, and youthful members, were evident, reflecting widening divisions in general society. When elders denounced the young people in their congregation for being sexually loose and frivolous, young men retorted that 'Elderly men are the problem. They preach to us about morals, while they swallow the girls and spoil them for us. We don't have money. When we do marry, our wives are already infected'. Elderly men, on the other hand, accused the youth of being careless and apathetic. They expressed shock at the way young boys laughed off HIV/ AIDS infection as an 'accident on the job' (*ajali kazini*), or their rationale that 'the sharp sting of bees never stopped people from getting honey' (*pamoja na ukali wa nyuki hauzui watu kufuata asali*). The youth were considered a 'lost generation, infiltrated by satanic attitudes and behaviour'. On their part, youth complained that their specific interests were not taken seriously in the church. They expressed alienation and powerlessness, and found the existing activities which were open to them to be limited and irrelevant (e.g. singing and running Sunday schools).

   Gender divisions were also surfacing in church circles. The HIV/AIDS epidemic provoked women to articulate an anger that had long festered. Women spoke with fury in all the discussion groups (both mixed and women alone) about the promiscuous sexual practices of men outside of marriage, and their selfishness and cunning in trying to hide unfaithfulness from their wives. According to these highly religious women, when men discovered that they were infected with HIV/AIDS, they suddenly pretended to be extra fine husbands so as not to lose their wives. Unmarried men with AIDS quickly found a 'good nice girl' to marry, innocent as to their status. As one woman said at a focus group discussion in Katumba village:

> All that is to make sure there is someone to take care of them when HIV/ AIDS is advanced. When they begin purging with diarrhoea and vomiting in bed, men badly need someone to look after them. Doing the washing of clothes soiled with faeces, bedpans, and dressing them with nappies, it

requires someone who really loves you and is highly committed. Who else but a wife, for the wife is bound by the marriage contract? For Christians, the marriage vows stipulate clearly that 'they will abide together in sickness and in health, until death separates them'. Such men exploit this for their selfish ends.

(Woman, Katumba village)

Even religious women insisted that they would not give in to such expectations, and would divorce their husbands instead, explaining that this was their response to male oppression. Why should they encourage other women to continue 'nappy changing' the men? Seropositive men would infect their wives; they would bring poverty to the household because a wife caring for a sick husband would not be able to farm or work properly; and they would disgrace the entire family so that their daughters remain unmarried. However, the cases of a wife actually divorcing a seropositive husband were rare.

The labour cost of caring for the sick has been given inadequate attention by AIDS prevention and support groups. The emotional as well as the economic impact should be more fully recognised (Barnett and Blaikie, 1992; Tibaijuka, 1997; Mbilinyi-Segule, 1999). In a discussion group in Ikama village, an elderly woman deplored the amount of 'precious time spent caring for our children, sick with AIDS'. Despite this, most families insisted on bringing patients home from the hospital, because of their distrust of hospital treatment. 'Once they know it is HIV/AIDS, they will not treat a person, they will just let her die'. An unlimited supply of labour and good will for caring cannot be taken for granted, however. Family systems may well have reached overload.

On the other hand, forms of collective caring provided some relief outside of the family, often within the context of the churches. The most notable was that of *kitulano*, the women's support groups of the Moravian church. Several instances were observed where *kitulano* groups voluntarily hoed a woman's field or harvested her crops when she was too weak to manage on her own. Members took turns providing water and firewood. According to Christian ethics, people ill with HIV/AIDS could not be 'dropped'. To be Christian is to have compassion and love (*huruma na upendo*).

Christians should also be forgiving. It was the devil who inflicted disaster (*shetani ameleta maafa*); the individual was therefore not responsible for having become infected and should be loved, not expelled or abjected. Carers urged sufferers to have faith in God, to 'ask God to forgive your sins', and be 'happy in your faith'. After someone had passed away, *kitulano* members along with others in the Christian community provided contributions in cash and kind for the funeral.

AIDS prevention: local struggles

The top leadership of the Moravian church in Rungwe deplored the use of condoms, and denounced them as vehicles of Western decadence, encouraging an indiscriminate sexual freedom neither traditional nor consistent with Christian morality. A 'nationalistic' discourse was thus used to delegitimise not only condoms, but young people with education who dared to challenge the authority of the church and its leaders.

Alternative interventions were proposed by the churches: repentance and faithfulness would stop the infection. Drawing on Ephesians 6: 11, young women Pentecostalists preached that spiritual powers provided their main weapon against the devilish disease. 'Repentance to a merciful God, prayer for forgiveness, will lead to victory over the enemy. God will provide spiritual armour to fight the disease'.

Some church leaders pitted the church and its congregation of believers against the state. For example, a Lutheran Bishop in Rungwe argued that, 'the government encourages people to commit adultery by encouraging them to use condoms, and uses educated people for this end'. He also denounced sex education for encouraging children into sexual intercourse, a common view among many church members. Tutors at the Lutengano seminary argued that the task of educating young people about 'responsible sexual practices' should be left in the hands of the church and the family, and was not the business of government.

In focus group discussions among male and female students at Kipoke secondary school, the church's banning of condoms was mentioned as one of the major reasons for the continued spread of AIDS. It is unlikely that young boys, and especially girls, will be able to access condoms and information about their use, until the present domination of church leaders over people's minds and behaviour is challenged. Even grown men explained that it was impossible to acquire condoms in more remote rural villages, due to the 'surveillance' of church leaders, church elders and ordinary members (in this case, Moravians). The dogmatic stand of the Christian church denies its members the right to make their own choices and to protect their lives.

Not all religious leaders, staff and lay members shared the dominant view – or at least they entertained doubts. In Rungwe, some Lutheran leaders and counsellors took a more ambiguous, if not positive, stand on HIV prevention. These local church leaders might not openly promote condoms, but they did not denounce their use. It is noteworthy that Lutheran hospitals distribute condoms free. For Catholics there were similarly mixed messages.[4] Such ambiguity offers a space in which discussion around condoms can focus more on safety than on sin. Such discussions expose gender and generational tensions.

Many women were not only anxious that men used condoms, but in case of male resistance they wondered whether there were no female condoms? In group discussions, other women explained that such condoms existed and were being sold in Tunduma – though for nearly two hundred and fifty times the price of a male condom. Women demanded that less expensive female condoms be made available, or that government distribute them free of charge. Whilst some women raised doubts about condoms, on the whole they were more positive about their use than men. Male elders tended to take a hard line, totally opposed to condom use in and out of marriage. Condoms conflicted with procreation – how would people bear children? Moreover, condom use would enable women to conduct extramarital affairs without their husbands' knowledge.

Unsurprisingly then, several women said that they were unable to raise the subject of condoms with their husbands/partners. When asked whether wives could demand that their husbands use a condom, nearly all replies were negative:

It's not normal according to tradition for women to decide, in fact, she'll be accused of being a prostitute.

She can use her powers of persuasion, but it is not easy.

Women are afraid of a quarrel. The man will protest, 'What are you accusing me of? Being a prostitute?'

Some misgivings about condoms were shared among women and men in focus group discussions: young men might lose their fertility if they did not ejaculate freely and often; condoms break; condoms have already been infected with the virus by 'outsider'/western interests. People also believed that condoms spoiled sexual pleasure – in the words of young people, it was like 'bathing in raincoats'. These views reflected the prevalence of a male model of sexual pleasure, associated with penetration, though some male elders spoke of alternative forms of male relief without ejaculating 'in' the woman. Different modes of experiencing sexual pleasure and satisfying desire among women were not discussed. These findings confirm those of research not only in Tanzania, but worldwide (Holland *et al.*, 1992; Baylies and Bujra, 1999).

Compared with villagers, well-to-do male traders and civil servants travelling through the area were more likely to use condoms in sexual relations outside of marriage. The owner of a prosperous local inn noted that his male clients openly demanded condoms on arrival, saying 'they (local women) want to kill me *(wataka mimi nife)*'. Free condoms were supplied in each room and were used.

Maria, a young bar maid employed at the same hotel, a primary school leaver aged 23 years and unmarried, said:

I learned about AIDS in class 7 and know all the symptoms. Hotel clients use condoms; the hotel knows because every time they check the rooms, they find the supply exhausted. The men want condoms; when they are used up they demand more. Before I marry, I will insist that my man gets an HIV check. If he is infected, there will be no wedding. My late mother told me about AIDS, and now I, in turn, caution my younger sister. For myself, I always use condoms when having sexual relations with men. Why do some women get AIDS? They take chances with their partners, not sure of their AIDS status. Moreover, some girls go with seropositive men because of money. But I will never do this. If men refuse to wear condoms, women should wear female condoms that should be distributed free to all.

(Maria, aged 23)

In general, single women were considered far more empowered than married women in relation to sex. They could legitimately refuse or negotiate condom use. In a discussion group with sex workers and bar maids in Katumba, some argued that they 'did not perform sex with just anybody'; and they insisted on using condoms. Only one barmaid had reportedly died of HIV/AIDS in the village, compared with many deaths amongst 'good married women'. Even sex workers were caught in a dilemma, however, as men paid more for unsafe sex.

Women in general displayed an extremely high level of distrust of men as well as a healthy instinct for self-preservation. When asked in interviews, 'What should someone do if they suspect or know that their partner is sero-positive?' they reported that:

Condoms can break – you'll be caught by lightening. Divorce is the only answer.

If it's my husband, I'll continue to live with him without any sexual intercourse.

This is a difficult situation – if it's a man, he'll marry another wife.

Men can't restrain themselves – better to divorce.

Condoms? He might take it off or tear it.

Examples were given of women who had refused to have sex with their partners, and sometimes succeeded in getting them tested for HIV, and of women who were allowed to divorce after it was found that the husband was seropositive. Conversely, there were seropositive men who told their friends and relatives that they would not die alone, that they would make sure their wives were also infected, lest they remain behind and 'profit'. Men's wilful transmission of the disease to their spouses was said to be proven by the number of men who died, followed by their wives and children. Only occasionally did one hear of exceptions, such as the two men in the neighbourhood who told their wives about their seropositive status, and abstained from sexual relations with them so that 'at least one of the parents would survive and care for the children'.

Men were much less likely to contemplate divorce than women if their wives became infected. More powerful than women, they are able to control sexual practices by protecting themselves – or acquiring another wife to meet their needs. Women lacked such options; their only safety lay in physical separation.

Concluding remarks

In this chapter, we have examined how Rungwe people are coping with a new hazard, HIV/AIDS, in the context of ongoing systemic changes (globalisation, monetisation, the decline in smallholder farming and changes in the gender division of labour). A variety of existing discourses were used to interpret the phenomenon of HIV/AIDS, in particular Christianity and notions of 'tradition'.

AIDS discourse is riddled with examples of scapegoating, if not demonising groups who have already been marginalised. Promiscuous men and women, independent women of any kind, but also now men in general are stigmatised as irresponsible, lazy and drunkards. These stereotypes – for that is what they have become – contribute to the construction of a powerful ideological imagery which blames the victims, and deflects attention away from basic causes. Whitehead (1999) has written of a long line of colonial and racist imagery about the lazy African, the drunken African, the promiscuous African (see also Mbilinyi, 1989). The fact that many married women, especially those in middle and elder age groups, profess such views towards errant men and women in their midst illustrates the power of such ideology.

One of the outstanding observations to be made on this basis of this study is the extent to which rural women in Rungwe have acquired greater independent power and control over economic activities and incomes in recent times, in a general context of growing impoverishment. Structures of male domination are threatened by the growing dependence of rural households on the cash incomes of women, be they poor or rich. This has occurred in part because of the reversal of fortunes for men, who have experienced a steady decline in farm incomes, wage incomes and formal wage employment. These developments have been reinforced by structural adjustment and liberalisation policies, which have undermined the sustainability of smallholder farming and livestock-keeping. The growing autonomy of women has consequences for their greater sexual freedom, but also portends their greater risk.

Despite the greater economic empowerment of women and the disempowerment of men, many married women are still powerless to demand safer sex, or to assert their own sexual needs. Perhaps distinctions need to be made between the expansion of women's income-earning activities and income *per se,* and men's continuing control over productive assets such as land, farm inputs and labour, in exploring the meaning, and limits, of 'economic power' in its impact on intimate relations. We also suspect a lag between transformation in economic conditions, and changes in ideology and sexual practice, especially within the confines of the household/family and the Christian 'community'.

Use of the condom is the main preventive measure being promoted by the National AIDS Control Programme, NGOs and the mass media, through social marketing campaigns and sensitisation workshops. A behavioural model of free choice is constructed, putting the onus on individual women and men to make the right choice – be it abstention, faithfulness or condoms. Condom use was promoted by AIDS counsellors in Rungwe, even those working within health facilities owned by religious institutions, and condoms were distributed free or at low cost by social marketing programmes. Yet existing gender constructions of sexual practice meant that most men rejected condoms and many women lacked the power to demand their use. Moreover, the major religious institutions preached against the condom. They promoted faithfulness in marriage, celibacy beforehand, and abstinence in cases of seroprevalence, which under present circumstances could only lead to female powerlessness and death.

Patriarchal constructions of marriage and family need to be challenged at all levels and within different spheres, including religion. There is an urgent need to analyse the construction of masculinities (see, for example, Mziray, 1998; Foreman, 1999; Rweyemamu, 1999; Bujra, 2000c). Without men, asserts Foreman, there would be no epidemic; whilst Schoepf (1997: 321) argues that, 'the AIDS epidemic will diminish as men come to terms with their own risks, accept responsibility to protect others, and change their sexual behaviour'. At the same time we should not forget that women are also active agents. These issues are complex and their investigation requires the use of tools of analysis from political economy, gender and cultural studies and psychology.

Socio-economic factors – migrant labour, white settler farming, racial policies in the colonial days, and more recently, the impact of economic liberalisation – have helped to shape AIDS along with gender relations (Bassett and Mhloyi, 1991; Barnett and Blaikie, 1992; Schoepf, 1997; Webb, 1997; Madunagu, 1998). Holistic studies are needed of historical changes in gender relationships, which locate sexual practice within the wider context of political, economic and ideological changes, conflicts and resistances. Ultimately, AIDS programmes need to engage with 'big questions' such as income inequalities, debt crisis, globalisation and the impoverishment of the majority (O'Malley, 1996).

Notes

1   The field research on which this chapter is based was carried out in Rungwe District in 1995–96 by Naomi Kaihula, assisted by David Mwaipopo. More detailed information can be found in Kaihula (1996a–c). Marjorie Mbilinyi wrote the chapter on the basis of information provided in field notes, reports and discussions with Naomi Kaihula, and drawing on her own earlier work in the area (Mbilinyi, 1989, 1991,

1997; Kalindile and Mbilinyi, 1991). She is grateful to the Cross Cultural Centre for Research on Women, Queen Elizabeth House, Oxford University, for a hospitable environment in which to write. The authors are appreciative of comments made on earlier reports by the Gender/AIDS group in Dar es Salaam and grateful to Janet Bujra and Carolyn Baylies for comments and continual support. Special thanks to the communities and institutions of Rungwe who participated in the field research.

2   The unusual degree of women's economic empowerment in Rungwe is emphasised by a comparison with Lushoto (Chapter 7). In Rungwe, 46 per cent of the women sampled in our base-line survey were self-employed (usually in trading) whilst 30 per cent were wage workers (the categories overlap for some). In Lushoto only 14 per cent were self-employed and 6 per cent in wage work. A case similar to that of Rungwe, with increasing female autonomy and sexual freedom, is to be found in neighbouring Kyela district (Aggleton and Warwick, 1999: 76).

3   This was in conjunction with a prevention and education programme organised by an NGO from Germany.

4   Whilst the Catholic church has prohibited the use of condoms, the work of Joinet (1994a,b) and his colleagues is distinctively different. It recognises all the different ways of preventing AIDS, without demonising any particular one. Abstinence or faithfulness would be best, but for those who cannot maintain these practices, use a condom! In Rungwe, a counsellor at a Roman Catholic facility confided that he surreptitiously gave condoms as well as advice on how to use them to his clients, in spite of the official church position. Joinet (1994a) has openly accused the church of being unfaithful to the call of Christ, in its casting out as devils or sinners those who have AIDS. Stigmatisation is 'anti-Christian', according to this outlook.

5 AIDS in Kanyama: contested sexual practice and the gendered dynamics of community interventions

Carolyn Baylies, Tashisho Chabala and Faustina Mkandawire

In exploring how AIDS is experienced and confronted in Kanyama, an urban neighbourhood in Zambia's capital, Lusaka; this chapter addresses a set of interrelated factors: a plurality of cultural backgrounds of residents; proximity to government, donor and NGO resources; deep poverty; and high levels of HIV vulnerability. With reference to these it considers two major issues.

The first is the way in which ideas about sexual behaviour are both informed by 'traditional' beliefs and practices[2] and in process of reconstruction, given a mixture of differing traditions, access to new information and, particularly, the impact of AIDS. A traditionalist discourse is typically invoked in attempts to preserve power relations which 'new ways of doing things' threaten to displace. In practice, the content of what passes for 'traditional' is never static but constantly articulating with 'new' ideas. Nevertheless the strong influence of 'past practices' and the moral logic which underlay them is evident in the way people seek to understand AIDS. But so too is a process of reflection and re-evaluation in attempts to come to terms with the danger which AIDS poses.

The second issue relates to the way interventions around AIDS have been experienced in Kanyama and the gender and class dynamics which have informed them. The neighbourhood's very proximity to the seat of government, donor and NGO operations has entailed a much higher level of activity there (and across Lusaka more generally) than elsewhere in the country. A considerable number of local residents have been trained, visited by home care teams and received peer education. Yet this very proximity to resources can magnify frustration when expectations are not fully met, co-ordination of efforts remains elusive or initiatives appear insufficiently supported. Aspirations toward communal benefit can also be undermined when 'community' programmes render a greater share of material rewards to those already relatively privileged and, although women give disproportionately of their time and effort, they receive less in respect of compensation or social prestige.

These two issues are brought together through a focus on a group of women in Kanyama who called themselves traditional educators, but were in fact drawn from various Christian denominations. They offered guidance to adolescent girls, prospective brides and married women on sexual matters, hygiene and marital relations. The content of their advice represented a mixture of Christian values and pre-existing cultural beliefs, which in the context of AIDS was undergoing further modification. They were one of a number of groups within Kanyama involved in work around AIDS and were enthusiastic about an initiative to achieve greater co-ordination through securing external support. As will be seen, the failure of this effort led to demoralisation and a contraction of their activities.

AIDS in Kanyama

Kanyama is a residential district of greater Lusaka, located about 2 km south of the city centre. It is composed of two sections, Old and New Kanyama. Old Kanyama mushroomed, unplanned, as a squatter settlement during the colonial period. It is the poorer part, characterised by higher density and smaller dwellings of inferior construction, piles of rubbish, few water taps, inadequate drainage, poor sanitation and ill-planned roads. In the early 1990s, there were about 36,000 people living in the area. New Kanyama, with a population of about 29,000, was originally established as a site and service scheme. As was customary with such projects, roads were laid out, water and street lighting provided, and plots demarcated. However, given rapid increases in population, amenities became inadequate. The relatively few water taps were sometimes commandeered by young men who charged water collectors by the bucket. Women reported having to get up as early as 1am to go searching for water, from leaking pipes, trenches or the community's taps. They could sometimes spend many hours in queues, having left their children, and often those ill with HIV or AIDS, at home.[3]

Kanyama has a health centre and there are two basic schools within its boundaries as well as a number of churches. The place is alive with activity and people are on the streets both night and day. A great deal of commerce goes on within Kanyama – in its markets, shops, bars and guest houses. Some residents are relatively well off and in the midst of general poverty there are large homes, often enclosed by walls. However bad the roads may be, there are some with not one but several cars. Jane and Sam, the couple whose situation is described in Box 5.1 are an example of those residents with relatively high incomes. Whether rich or poor, no one escapes the threat of AIDS.

> ## Box 5.1 Case study of a discordant couple in Kanyama
> ## by Faustina Mkandawire
>
> I first met Jane (not her real name) on 18 March 1996, the very day that she had an HIV test. My research colleagues and I asked if we could include her in our survey and she agreed. After completing the questionnaire, she asked if we would return to speak to her husband. She was

very worried that he might be infected with HIV. When we returned to the house on 22 March 1996, we found Sam at home alone. This gave us an opportunity to talk about the research we were doing and about the problem of AIDS in the community. Jane came back from town while we were still there. As we were all talking together, the issue of using condoms came up. They had used condoms throughout their marriage for contraception, but Sam complained that they were now 'burning' him and said he did not want to continue using them. We then talked about how families are affected when parents are at loggerheads about condoms and discussed their reactions, were they to discover that one or both of them was HIV positive. At the end of the session both Sam and Jane seemed happy that a number of issues had been aired that they would have felt uncomfortable discussing on their own.

When we met them, Sam and Jane had been married for 21 years. Both had reached grade seven in school. Sam used to work in a bank in Lusaka, but now owned a bar, several houses and a number of cars. Jane was running her own business buying and selling clothing. They had eight children, the oldest aged 21 and the youngest just 5 years old. They were also looking after three other girls orphaned by AIDS. Two were daughters of Sam's sister and the other was the daughter of Jane's cousin. Sam had had many girlfriends both before and during his marriage. Jane used to confront them and beat them up, but then one day decided that she would only lose her life if she continued chasing Sam's girlfriends. So she stopped behaving like a 'mad woman', as she put it. She just minded her own business but at the same time made sure she protected herself from AIDS.

Several years ago, Sam became very ill and nearly died. Nobody thought he would recover. Jane nursed him day and night at the hospital. When his relatives saw how ill he was, they started sharing out the family's property. This hurt Jane deeply, since none had even helped with his care. With the assistance of her own relatives, Jane intervened to prevent the property grabbing. Sam recovered enough to be discharged and Jane continued to nurse him at home, but he frequently suffered new bouts of illness and once was diagnosed with T.B.

When Sam suggested to Jane that they stop using condoms and try for another child, Jane expressed her misgivings, saying that the house was full. She then suggested that they both go and have HIV tests, just to make sure that they were negative. She secretly worried that Sam's frequent illnesses might be a sign that he was HIV-positive. The death of her sister-in-law added to worries about her own health. She had been having problems with her legs for some time, to the extent of finding it difficult to walk. If both she and Sam were to die, who would support their children and their orphaned relatives? So Jane decided to go for the test.

Sam did not go with her. Displeased about her not wanting to stop using condoms, he acquired another girlfriend, who soon became pregnant. Sam stopped supporting his family and Jane had to struggle to feed and keep her children in school. All the while Sam continued to harass Jane about the condom issue and even accused her of having a boyfriend. That was the reason, he claimed, that she did not want to stop using condoms. Sam and Jane frequently quarrelled. Sam also scolded the children who, in turn, took their hurt and frustration out on one another, especially the youngest.

Jane went alone to get her test results. They were negative, but another test was arranged for the beginning of August. Sam did not enquire about the test results and Jane concluded that he did not care about her health. So she decided not to tell him. Within 2 weeks Sam was ill again and Jane had to take him to the hospital where an HIV test was done. It was positive. Despite pre-counselling, Sam took the result badly, tearing up the form and accusing Jane of bribing the doctors because she wanted him to leave his girlfriend. She told him he could go wherever he liked, if that was what he wanted. That very day Sam left for his girlfriend's house. In the presence of his friends he asked his girlfriend if she felt at all ill. She said she was all right. Sam then turned to his friends, asking how come the girlfriend who is pregnant is all right but he is said to be HIV positive by the doctor? His relatives then ordered Jane not to take Sam anywhere when he got sick without their permission.

Sam continued to deny that he was HIV positive and discouraged his girlfriend from taking a test. When I stopped by their house in early August 1996, Jane said Sam was still harassing her over the condom issue. She was clearly very distressed and had got to the point of telling him that she herself was positive and asking if he wanted to get the virus from her. She had come to fear that Sam would kill her during the night and therefore would only go to bed once he was asleep. Their use of the same toilet also became a cause for worry. She was even afraid of touching his body at night because he was sweating a lot and the fluid made her feel unsafe. However, gradually her fears for herself subsided and she became worried about Sam. He had begun to have diarrhoea and an X-ray showed spots on his lungs. He was reluctant to go for treatment as the doctor had advised. She had tried to contact his relatives for permission to take him to hospital, but without success.

At least Sam had renewed his relationship with his children and was no longer quarrelling as often with Jane. He was becoming forgetful, however, and Jane feared that he was losing his mind. When he had any leftovers on his plate he would hide them and occasionally became very angry without cause. The couple had been referred to an NGO in Lusaka which provided counselling. Jane felt that the children also need counselling.

Poverty generated other environments of risk. The struggle for survival of many in Kanyama is evident from the tiny stalls outside their homes where small packets of rice or sugar or other goods are on sale, the sorry state of their dwellings and the malnourished appearance of children on the street. Many families had meals only once a day.[4] The notion of shared poverty – with meagre income redistributed through the selling of goods and services – has stark meaning in this neighbourhood where relatively little generation of new value is evident. The extent to which the exchange of sexual favours is not just a 'survival strategy' but routinised as an accessory to other commercial transactions is revealed by claims that casual sex goes on in shops with girls 'going for young men' who can facilitate access to the groceries sold there.[5]

It has been estimated that as many as 60 per cent of households in Kanyama may be headed by women (Hughes-d'Aeth, 1998). Box 3 depicts the situation of three women, two on their own and one still married, albeit tenuously. While many are capable and strong, the position of others is precarious. Those with children and few means for feeding them sometimes turn to sex work. Given their alienation from even the possibility of wage labour, they have little to sell save their capacity to engage in sex.

Box 5.2 Three women: the divorcee, the wife, and the widow – from the research diary of Tashisho Chabala

7 February 1996 – the divorcee, cashier in a bar
Mary had three children, aged 10, 8 and 6, and had been divorced since 1989. She was currently seeing a man she had met in the bar where she worked. She felt he was honest and would make a good husband. She told me she had many friends in the same business as she was. Most were unmarried, but had boy-friends who provided them with most of the things they needed. Some of her friends had died after suffering from swelling of the legs, malaria, T.B. and diarrhoea. She had no doubt that they died of AIDS because of the symptoms and the many sexual partners they had had. After observing these deaths, many of those still alive had resorted to using condoms which they bought themselves.

Mary accused men of abandoning their wives when they got a bit of money and 'going for' prostitutes. Ironically, this had been the reason for her own divorce. Her former husband had been 'sleeping out' (i.e. not coming home at night) for some 3 months before they parted. 'Why should a poor woman suffer for the sins of an irresponsible husband?' she asked. 'He should be left to pay for his sins'.

8 February 1996 – the married women, a seller of charcoal
Helen was married with six children, and also looking after two nieces whose parents died of T.B. the previous year. She complained of severe economic hardship. The family had moved to Kanyama when her husband was sacked 3 years earlier. After 1 year his redundancy money was gone and she had had to start selling charcoal. The marriage was on the rocks, mainly because her husband was constantly grabbing money from her for drinking and frequently 'sleeping out'. She knew he had girl-friends in drinking places. Life was difficult, she said. She had supported many women who had left their husbands. 'When a woman goes through an experience like mine, what can prevent her from leaving her husband?' she asked.

13 January 1996 – the widow, a brewer of beer
On my way back to the market place, I passed by two houses where *kachasu* was brewed. There were men drinking at both, even though it was only 10 o'clock in the morning. A quarrel had erupted between a married couple at the second house, with the wife accusing her husband of having neglected his family by 'sleeping out' for the previous 2 weeks. She wanted to fight the woman who was selling *kachasu*, whom she suspected of sleeping with her husband. She was worried about being infected with HIV and threatened to 'do something' if she got AIDS. She accused the woman selling *kachasu* – a widow whose own husband had died 3 years earlier – of having killed a lot of men by infecting them with HIV and implored her husband not to bring the 'disease' home. So distraught was she that a friend had to lead her away.

As the two women left, another who was watching the scene said, 'this is a disgrace for us single women brewing *kachasu*. Everyone will be thinking that we are destroying peoples' marriages'. I asked her what should be done, but she answered that there was nothing. She just wished people (especially men) respected their own families and avoided extra-marital affairs. 'The problem with men', she said, 'is that they don't even fear AIDS'. I asked what she would do to protect herself from being infected if she were in the wife's shoes. She replied, 'if I die of AIDS that means that is how my death was to come. There is nothing I can do'.

Since she was going to the market, we walked together. On the way she told me that she felt pity for the woman selling *kachasu* and I sympathised with her. Her own husband, she said, died 2 years previously. She was sure he died of AIDS, for she knew that he had been with other women. She had been unable to protect herself. 'I was worried about losing my marital status and my children. I had to just stay in marriage'. She wished condoms had been widely publicised at that time. She has five children.

Kanyama is a lively but also a dangerous place to live. The level of crime is high and shootings are not uncommon. Its population is a mixture of people from most parts of Zambia as well as further afield; some are transient; some come precisely for the 'night life' on offer, with the 'guest' houses' being populated, especially on the weekends, by visiting 'businessmen'.

Data from the small survey which we carried out in the early months of 1996 can only be taken as indicative, but provides some insight concerning the social composition and views of residents. Only a small minority (14 per cent) were born locally and thus 'from' Kanyama. In terms of ethnicity and language group, 15 per cent were Ngoni or Chewa, 14 per cent Kaonde or Ila, 14 per cent Bemba, 10 per cent Tumbuka and 10 per cent Tonga, with smaller proportions from a range of other groups. This diversity was evident in focus group discussions where establishing a *lingua franca* sometimes proved diffi-cult, underlining the larger challenges of establishing communal cohesive-ness.

AIDS was readily acknowledged as a problem within the community. Estimates of adult prevalence applying to Lusaka as a whole for 1997, at 30 per cent, confirm the severity of the situation (Ministry of Health, Zambia, 1997). According to a traditional birth attendant working in the community, while many sought care at the clinic or at Lusaka's University Teaching Hospital, others died quietly in their homes due to lack of transport money and inability to pay the fees.[6] People registered the depth of the problem in the number of deaths:

A lot of people have died; some are sick. My son died.

A number of people are dying. I have just come from a burial.

Many people have died from AIDS.

(Kanyama survey respondents)[7]

Kanyama market had a special committee for organising funerals of people sell-ing there; in the mid 1990s there was a funeral nearly once a fortnight.[8]

About 70 per cent of both male and female respondents felt themselves to be in danger from AIDS, although a higher proportion of women than men said that AIDS had had a direct impact on their lives.[9] Women were also more prone to say that AIDS had increased gender conflict within the community.[10] However, a majority of both men and women concurred that tension had increased: 'it has brought confusion in homes; there is much mistrust'.[11] Almost two-fifths of the sample said that they had heard of cases of marriage break-up instigated by HIV/AIDS, often with gender-specific terminology referring to husbands divorcing wives, as against wives 'running away':

> When the husband became critically sick, the wife just ran away.

> Here in Kanyama, the wife left her husband because he showed symptoms of HIV/AIDS.

> My friend divorced his wife because he suspected her of having had sex with a man who was believed to be infected.[12]

All this presents a picture of pain, dislocation, resentment and enormous hardship, both for those immediately involved as well as their relations and dependants. Many children in Kanyama have been orphaned, and some of these have ended up on the streets, in turn highly vulnerable to HIV infection.

AIDS and sexual practices: reconstructing ideas about sexuality and vulnerability

In striving to understand how and why infection occurs, people in Kanyama drew on a medical discourse communicated through health education messages as well as on deeply ingrained views about sex and blood as life forces and transgressions associated with sexual behaviour leading to ill health. Focus groups became occasions where participants explored their views against the contrasting interpretations of others. A prominent theme was the question of whether AIDS was a new or old disease. Most regarded AIDS as different because incurable, but sometimes boundaries were blurred. One participant in a male focus group, for example, linked HIV infection with 'older' ideas about sex at improper times. Were he to have sex with someone who had had an abortion, he said, sores would appear on his body:

> This is because the woman's blood is rotten. You see, we exchange the blood. She takes mine and I take hers. When I take hers I will get infected and she will also get infected.

This, he said, would 'turn into' HIV infection. He then turned to the case of a stillbirth. Were he to have sex with his wife after this event, this would also 'cause' HIV infection. He explained how such outcomes could be prevented:

> We should wait for the woman to recover before starting having sex. This

should be done like in the olden days. The lady had to have her periods two or three times before the husband had sex with her. The blood was then considered to be 'clean'. This is what causes sickness in men.[13]

There may be many versions of 'traditional' illnesses, applying among different groups and understood in different ways. Our concern here, however, is with how people make sense of them and of AIDS in respect of them. What was common to most (and similar to what was described in the case of Kapulanga in Chapter 3) was their formulation in respect of women's bodies, portraying women as being unclean and men as susceptible to illness by engaging – knowingly or not – in sexual behaviour with such women at such times.

Miscarriages or abortions were most commonly regarded as the basis for triggering such illnesses, but reference was also in made in Kanyama to young girls not observing certain customs after 'coming of age'[14], or, to a 'very sexy' woman reaching her orgasm before her partner did.[15] Illness afflicting men was also associated with women's failure to observe taboos against cooking, or sometimes even against adding salt to relish, during their menstrual periods or after childbirth.[16] On this basis some believed that HIV could be contracted by eating food sold in the market or on the street[17] and thus saw the epidemic as propelled by commerce as well as by sexual transgressions.

What troubled some people (particularly older people) was the lack of observance of cleansing rituals, that is, the failure to observe tradition. As one said:

In those days a woman would be advised not to sleep with her husband after a miscarriage. She had to wait for some time until she was cleansed. These customs are never observed in modern societies.

(Kanyama focus group)[18]

Another concurred: 'that is why AIDS in Zambia is spreading. We do not correct the children'.[19] In the wider context of such views, AIDS was seen not so much as a punishment for transgression against custom and moral precepts (though some certainly believed it to be) but more straightforwardly as its logical consequence.

That such ideas are drawn upon, but also debated and contested, however, is illustrated by the following exchange within a focus group discussion involving adolescent males:

In my opinion AIDS is transmitted through having sex with a girl or woman who has had either a miscarriage or an abortion. From what I hear, a person who has slept with such a woman will show all the symptoms as that of an HIV/AIDS person.

No. HIV/AIDS is basically an effect of indulgence in unprotected, extra-marital sex. In fact it results from promiscuity.

(Kanyama focus group)[20]

As well as debate over whether AIDS was new or old, a consequence of disregard of specific customs or of a more general promiscuity, there was also contention over the role of particular sexual practices in relation to HIV transmission. A case in point was dry sex, involving women's use of various techniques to dry and tighten the vagina, sometimes in the belief that it had hygienic benefits, but primarily as a means of enhancing men's pleasure (Sandala *et al.*, 1995). As a participant in a men's focus group commented, 'when the liquid is too much, then the girl sees she has no value because men don't go back to her. Therefore, she thinks of medicine in order to be dry. Then the men also start coming to her'.[21] Some women also used drying techniques after childbirth. As one explained, 'after delivery, the 'way' is enlarged. Men don't like it that way'.[22] Sometimes a cloth was used for drying and sometimes herbs were inserted. However, a common method used in Kanyama involved drinking a porridge made from powders and roots: 'this trade is well known. When you find women gathered at a home, just know that it is medicine'.[23]

The extent of the threat posed by this practice remains unclear (Hira *et al.*, 1990; Sandala *et al.*, 1995),[24] but worries that it can cause abrasions and thereby increase the probability of HIV transmission have led to warnings from AIDS awareness campaigners. In consequence it has become open to public examination. A member of a group of older women who offered their services as Christian traditional educators in matters of sexual health was adamant in her denunciation of the practice: 'in the olden days traditional educators told girls to wear, drink and bathe in medicine in order to keep the man because (by doing this) one would become dry and warm. If you encourage this now some get cut during sex. ... it is a good environment for HIV to be transmitted because the woman could get cut. ...When teaching the girls we must tell them to stop using these drying catalysts'.[25]

Not all the women in this group felt it possible to persuade women and girls to avoid the practice. Nor did they all subscribe fully to a medical view of AIDS as a new illness. However, they were convinced of the need to warn women and girls of the danger it implied. It is to a closer account of this group that we now turn.

Contribution of traditional educators to AIDS education

Traditional educators, sometimes called traditional marriage counsellors or *Bana Fimbusa*, are found throughout Zambia. They provide counselling and give advice during initiation ceremonies and just prior to marriage, but they also attempt to reconcile disputes within marriage. Most are women, but men sometimes educate as well, each sex generally dealing with their own.

The characteristic message to women has been one of accommodation to men's authority, desires and vagaries of behaviour. Although not the case with the Kanyama group,[26] they sometimes charge for their services and have been known to adjust the quality of their advice to the level of expected compensation.[27]

Each educator draws on the specific customs of his or her own ethnic group in teaching what is regarded as appropriate sexual behaviour and gender roles. But as Christianity is widespread in Zambia (in Kanyama 84 per cent of respondents to our survey said they were adherents) the advice of many of those who call themselves 'traditional' educators represented an intertwining of Christian and indigenous precepts. AIDS activists at national level and particularly NGOs such as the Society for Women and AIDS in Zambia, have directed particular attention to traditional educators, given the nature of their work. If uninformed, their guidance can sometimes be unhelpful, but, if trained, they can use their role to impart knowledge about HIV and means of protection (Mushinge and Simwanza, 1996; Sikanyika, 1996).

The group of Christian traditional educators with which the research team worked in Kanyama provides an example of the interplay of competing discourses and the dynamics of collective learning in the context of AIDS. Not only did they wish to guide adolescent females and their fellow women on a moral pathway incorporating those customs which they regarded as consistent with their religious beliefs, but they also operated in an urban, pluralist context of competing 'traditions' and amongst other traditional educators whose customs and advice they sometimes regarded as 'too traditional' or not sufficiently Christian. Thus, on attending initiation ceremonies, they would place money in a plate, as was customary for gaining the floor, and use the occasion to interpret the relevance of their Christian beliefs to a woman's sexual deportment both within and outside of marriage.[28] Having received training about AIDS they appreciated the necessity of incorporating prevention advice in their activities. In any case, they had seen its effects all around them. Several of them were widows. Most had a relative who had died of AIDS. Many had personally cared for those who were ill.

The group had emerged in the early 1970s, prior to the AIDS epidemic, out of concern about the marital difficulties experienced by members of their church congregations. On the basis of some initial instruction from a pastor's wife, they set themselves up as Christian educators. In the mid 1990s there were 23 women in this group in Kanyama, representing a range of ethnic groups and churches, and linked with Zambia's Christian Council of Churches. Individual members of the group had acquired different specialisations. Some offered advice to girls at puberty about how to manage their periods, instructed them on the dangers of STDs and the undesirability of pre-marital pregnancies and counselled them to respect their elders. Others offered instruction just prior to a wedding, touching on sexual behaviour and potential domestic problems. In the context of AIDS, their teaching had extended to include advice to young girls on how to 'say no to sex', instruction on HIV as well as STDs, advocacy of HIV testing for those intending to marry, advice on dealing with a husband who had other partners and training in the care of those with HIV or AIDS and the upbringing of orphans.[29]

They did not always realise success in their teaching. As one member acknowledged, when they left discussion of AIDS until just prior to marriage, girls did not 'listen to us because we did not tell them right from an early age'.[30] In consequence some felt it important to alert girls to the dangers of HIV much earlier. Yet few could countenance the teaching of precisely the same message at this age that they would give just prior to marriage. Theirs was still a doctrine of control and containment of adolescent urges:

> The lesson here is that we should adhere to the morals and culture and teach our children about AIDS.

The coupling of morals and culture was crucial. The core of their message was to counsel personal hygiene, respect for elders, and especially, as one put it: 'no sleeping with boys'. It would not do, in their view, to teach sexual techniques at, let alone before, puberty, since to do so would encourage immorality. Ironically, in the days when marriage followed soon after puberty, instruction in 'how to handle a man in bed' (as it was often described) occurred at this time. But now, with later marriage, some Christian educators were adamant that it should be deferred:

> A long time ago, our children used to grow without having sex with the opposite sex. But now even before she is mature she has already started. Therefore, at what stage should we start teaching these girls things of a home such as sex? Because if we teach them before puberty, maturity, they would put into practice the same lesson. We have to change our ways of teaching on sex. A child who reaches of age but is not ready for marriage should not be taught on the way a man is to be handled in bed. This disease is there because of lack of morals.[31]

The change in 'ways of teaching' followed a Christian logic, but in the context of AIDS could be problematic and other changes might be more appropriate.

Members of the group did not have equivalent levels of knowledge about HIV/AIDS and disagreed about precisely what should be taught when. That the nature of their advice was not always palatable to its recipients is evident from their dismay that young people often 'do not listen'.[32] But the depth of their anxiety about the deaths around them, not least of their children, made them eager to learn from health workers and incorporate this knowledge in their own teaching. As one member of the research team put it, theirs were modern eyes, attempting (albeit within boundaries set by their Christian belief) to see what was good (and bad) in the past, present and future.[33]

Community interventions around AIDS in Kanyama: successes and frustrations

The work of this group of church-based traditional educators is but one example of AIDS-related activity in Kanyama. Over the middle years of the decade there were a number of interventions, some specifically concerned with AIDS and others having an AIDS component. The most significant were a peer education programme supported by UNICEF and NORAD, a home based care programme operating under the auspices of the Catholic church and a set of projects run by CARE International, some of which were supported by the then ODA. In addition, several churches ran AIDS support programmes for their members.

To judge from answers in our survey, the best known among AIDS activists were the peer educators. This was a programme modelled on a similar initiative in another part of Lusaka, which targeted vulnerable women, including sex workers.[34] Peer educators wore distinctive T-shirts, worked in small, close-knit groups and moved around the area performing mini-dramas about AIDS, facilitating general discussion, and distributing condoms. In 1995, they numbered twelve women and one man and worked closely with the health centre.

The home based care programme under the Catholic church largely supplanted an earlier programme, which had operated under the auspices of the Kanyama clinic, but which by the mid 1990s had essentially ceased to exist.[35] The new initiative began in 1994 around a group of eight women who received training in counselling and care of those with HIV. Members visited homes throughout Kanyama, providing counselling on care and assistance, when possible, with transport. The programme subsequently expanded with members organised in small teams so as to be responsible for particular sections of the community. Food received via the World Food Programme, the EU and some private benefactors was provided where possible and care and education activities were undertaken. Of sixty volunteers in the summer of 1998, all but fifteen were women. While receiving no pay, they were issued with boots and umbrellas and were enrolled in a medical scheme.[36]

The international NGO, CARE, also ran a number of programmes which variously bore directly or indirectly on AIDS. In the mid 1990s CARE's activities were primarily concerned with poverty alleviation through means intended to build local capacity and encourage collective development efforts. The NGO facilitated the emergence of a Residents' Development Committee (RDC) based on a system of representation of residents in demarcated zones, whose function was to monitor local development activities. CARE also ran the Peri-urban Self Help (PUSH) programme, through which foodstuffs from the World Food Programme were distributed to those most in need (mainly women and often widows) in exchange for work in the community, primarily on projects such as resurfacing roads or garbage collection. PUSH workers received health education, including instruction in family planning, AIDS prevention and care of AIDS patients, as well as literacy training, and were encouraged to form groups through which to apply for loans for income generating endeavours. Twenty-two members of PUSH were also trained as traditional birth attendants (TBAs) and given additional training in the care and counselling of AIDS patients.[37] A number of community health workers were also trained.

In the mid 1990s, our research team encountered both high levels of commitment and evident frustration among those involved in AIDS work in Kanyama. Although a number of activities were ongoing, certain groups felt particularly frustrated by lack of support as well as limited co-ordination between their efforts and those of others. The Christian traditional educators, for example, received encouragement from their various churches. However, women in the group felt hampered by lack of funds. Rather than receive payment for their services, they often found themselves having to pay when attending an initiation ceremony in order to gain the floor and provide advice about AIDS. They felt isolated and wanted more contact with others doing related work. Most important they wanted more information. The health workers who had come to tell them about AIDS had left them with incomplete information: ' the nurses had told us that they would come back and teach us but they have never come back'.[38]

A possible means of further integration seemed to present itself in the form of a Health Neighbourhood Watch Committee (HNWC), which was initially established by the matron of Kanyama Health Centre to support its work. Its members were selected in a similar way to the Resident Development Committee, by residents within demarcated zones. It received some funding from the British Overseas Development Agency (ODA), and the Ministry of Health provided money to facilitate its meetings, but it had also been encouraged to apply for additional support for its projects. Avowedly non-political, its brief was to draw up an action plan to improve the health of Kanyama residents.

Towards the end of 1996, the research team helped to set up a meeting to explore the possibility of the HNWC taking on a larger role in co-ordinating AIDS activities within the community. It was attended by representatives from CARE's PUSH project, the RDC, traditional healers, traditional educators, the Health Neighbour Watch Committee, the and the Catholic church's home based care programme. Their discussion pointed to a number of areas where networking might indeed prove beneficial. Women in the various church groups were carrying out home visits but not notifying the health centre or the HNWC of pockets of need. The RDC routinely encountered health problems in its community development work and, though aware of the HNWC, did not know precisely whom to contact when required. Although traditional educators had no regular contact with the HNWC, the latter's representative observed that they could be easily and beneficially incorporated into zone-based activities.

The meeting generated enthusiasm for greater networking and the germ of a plan to bring the traditional birth attendants and the traditional educators under the umbrella of the Health Neighbourhood Watch Committee for the purpose of seeking external support for their activities from external bodies. Work progressed some distance in this regard. The head of the Society for Women and AIDS in Zambia indicated willingness to meet with the traditional educators and give them further training and support. However, most important was the keen interest shown by functionaries in the Ministry of Sport, Youth and Child Development to 'adopt' these two groups in a pilot project. Plans were set in motion to hold a workshop in a Lusaka hotel as a basis for further collaboration.

Yet ultimately these plans became mired in bureaucracy and frustrated by the departure from their posts, via promotions and more prestigious appointments, of key individuals. During this same time, the HNWC and the RDC were also beset by problems of goal displacement. In the event, the RDC was disbanded and a new committee elected, while the HNWC seems to have gradually become inert.[39]

By the summer of 1998, many of those who had been involved in the abortive networking initiative harboured a strong sense of frustration. The traditional educators were no longer operating as an ecumenical group, nor even as a collective entity. One of their most prominent members had become the vice chair of the Christian Council at provincial level. Another had received further training in home based care and benefitted from an 'incentive' payment as a workshop participant. Of the others, however, some were now charging for their services, some had stopped their work altogether because there was 'no benefit' and they would 'rather do a business of selling tomatoes from their homes', while others had withdrawn to their various churches. As one of the original group commented, they had returned to their congregations to serve as traditional educators because 'church activities reward people with recognition in society and respect, unlike other voluntary work'.[40]

Gender and class dynamics of AIDS work in Kanyama

Work around AIDS has continued in Kanyama, with new energies being drawn on and additional community members being touched by AIDS awareness messages. Although some initiatives continued to make productive impact, most notably the peer educators based at the health centre, there has been a pattern in Kanyama, as elsewhere, of energies, talents, training, enthusiasm and commitment sometimes being less well utilised than the crisis posed by AIDS demands. Even during the few years covered by this case study, there was evidence of programmes being started, inadequately supported, and poorly integrated with ongoing work, with many who had received specialised training no longer using their skills. Equally important, the collective learning observed earlier appeared in some cases to have stagnated. Not only had traditional educators gone back to their respective churches, but in some cases they had gone back to the way they previously taught.

There was sadness but also a certain bitterness about the failure of plans for networking and increased support to materialise. Some suspected that the research team had gobbled up the money which was thought to have been allocated to the planned workshop. Others believed that it had never been the intention to 'hand them on to the government'. Yet others felt that the research team was just interested in getting their knowledge and had then forgotten about them.[41]

However, the problems were deeper than those of aborted facilitative efforts by the research team and related to broader efforts (and failures) of NGOs, donors and the government. Some of the difficulties countered by both the RDC and HNWC, for example, related to attempts by politicians to gain control over local initiatives. As one of the leaders of the RDC commented in 1998, 'political interference has caused a lot of underdevelopment'.[42] The task that some NGOs and donors have undertaken of trying to build a genuine community base for local development activity may be admirable in its intentions and even far-sighted in trying initially to side-step but ultimately to bolster local government. But it may also be potentially hazardous in challenging the interests and patronage networks of local politicians. It is often such vested interests which ultimately prevail and are indeed pandered to (sometimes deliberately, sometimes inadvertently) by external actors.

There was also evidence of organisations in Kanyama being used for personal gain, to the detriment of broader objectives of assisting those affected by AIDS. The pattern of activity around AIDS in the community broadly replicated that of development work more generally in perpetuating and indeed exacerbating inequalities – ironically the very inequalities upon which AIDS 'feeds'. While many have been recipients of AIDS education and care, the number in need far exceeds those assisted. At the same time, the paid jobs in these programmes, and therefore the most sustained benefits, go disproportionately to those already relatively privileged. Top positions in the RDC and the HNWC were not always held by the most affluent members of the community and indeed RDC members complained in 1996 about lack of recognition of or compensation for their work. Even so, there was a tendency for prominent members of these groups to be businessmen (or occasionally business women), owners of fleets of taxis, salaried employees, owners of cars, and residents of some of the community's larger residences. Although they may have had a genuine wish to serve the community, their posts were also used for personal gain, as stepping stones to other rewards.

While women were certainly among those in paid posts (in the peer education programme, at the clinic, in the CARE office), far more striking was their over-representation among those who were 'volunteers' and who continued to care and to serve their neighbours for relatively little reward. Women predominated among peer educators and home based care workers. They also made up the ranks of traditional educators and birth attendants. Class and gender dynamics were thus bound up in the process of community management in ways which, if predictable, still need to be remarked on and critically appraised.

Conclusions

In Kanyama, the depth of the AIDS crisis causes great anxiety among residents. A process of collective learning is ongoing among community residents and especially among groups involved in AIDS work. But knowledge is often incomplete and messages sometimes fashioned by moral or religious conviction in ways which, while effective for some audiences, may be less so for others. Yet there was a willingness to learn and contribute more. Many were desperate to make an impact on the problem. Their bitterness was all the greater, therefore, when initiatives fell through or individuals seemed to hijack efforts or to use their positions for personal ends. Ironically, and in spite of attempts by donors and NGOs to mobilise democratic participation through committees elected by residents in demarcated zones, it was often those closest to the grass roots, highly committed and genuinely altruistic, who lost out. Not coincidentally these were often poorer, frequently less well educated and predominantly female. Those already relatively privileged tended to claim or gain what scarce resources and rewards were on offer, whether these were salaries, sitting allowances, or training. These dynamics are important to the struggle around AIDS, not least because their outcomes can be so dispiriting to those at the bottom, leading to disillusionment and a disinclination to sustain their activities.

Notes

1 This chapter is based on research carried out in Kanyama between September 1995 and March 1997, with a follow-up set of interviews conducted in June 1998. The research was overseen by Beatrice Liatto-Katundu and carried out by Faustina Mkandawire, Olive Munjanja, Tashisho Chabala, Augustine Mkandawire and John Zulu. As well as conducting a baseline survey of one hundred residents and carrying out interviews with a wide range of key informants, a series of focus group discussions were held.

2 This process has been noted by a number of writers, in Zambia, for example, by Mukonde (1992) and more generally by de Bruyn (1992).

3 Research diary, O. Munjanja, September 1995. Water was pivotal to community intervention activities and a cause of persistent anxiety.

4 Research diary, F. Mkandawire, 4 May 1998.

5 Research diary, T. Chabala, 7 February 1996.

6 Research diary, O. Munjanja, 20 September 1995.

7 Kanyama survey, 1996.

8 Research diary, T. Chabala, 6 February 1996.

9 The figures were 61 per cent of women and 34 per cent of men, representing a significant difference in views on this matter ($\chi^2 = 7.36$, d.f. = 1, $p = 0.01$).

10 This applied to 84 per cent of women and 61 per cent of men, a difference which is statistically significant ($\chi^2 = 6.2$, d.f. = 1, $p = 0.01$).

11 Kanyama survey respondents.
12 Kanyama survey respondents.
13 Kanyama focus group, RDC, 18 September 1996, facilitator F. Mkandawire.
14 Kanyama focus groups, women, traditional educators, September 1996, facilitator F. Mkandawire; traditional healers, 25 April 1996, facilitator A. Mkandawire.
15 Kanyama focus group, traditional healers, 25 April 1996, facilitator A. Mkandawire.
16 Kanyama focus group, women, traditional educators, September 1996, facilitator F. Mkandawire; RDC, 18 September 1996, facilitator F. Mkandawire.
17 Research diary, T. Chabala, 8 February 1996.
18 Women, 46 and above, April 96, facilitators, A. Mkandawire and F. Mkandawire.
19 Kanyama focus group, RDC, 17 September 1996, facilitator F. Mkandawire.
20 Men, 15–19, 25 April 1996.
21 Kanyama focus group, men, 21–45, 24 April 1996, facilitator, A. Mkandawire.
22 Kanyama focus group, women, 21–45, 24 April 1996, facilitator, A. Mkandawire.
23 Kanyama focus group, women, traditional educators, 13 September 1996, facilitator F. Mkandawire.
24 Hira *et al.*'s (1990) data suggested that the relative risk of HIV-1 infection was twenty-eight times greater among women using a cloth to remove vaginal secretions. Sandala *et al.* (1995), who investigated 'dry sex' in relationship to HIV infection, found little evidence of a strong connection but still concluded that women should still be counselled about its potential harm.
25 Kanyama focus group, women, traditional educators, 13 September 1996, facilitator, F. Mkandawire.
26 Members of the group emphasised the distinction between those traditional educators who charged for their services and themselves as not paid because they were 'from the church'. However, they did sometimes receive gifts of appreciation. (Kanyama focus group, females, traditional educators, 13 September 1996, facilitator, F. Mkandawire; Research diary, F. Mkandawire, March 1996).
27 Research diary, Mansa, T. Chabala, 24 May 1996.
28 Research diary, F. Mkandawire, March 1996; 20 December 1997.
29 Research diary, F. Mkandawire, March 1996; June 1998.
30 Kanyama focus group, traditional educators, 13 September 1996, facilitator F. Mkandawire.
31 Ibid.
32 Ibid.
33 Letter, F. Mkandawire, February 2000.
34 Interview, Lusaka, November 1995.
35 Research diaries, O. Munjanja, September 1995; T. Chabala, February 1996; F. Mkandawire, June 1998.
36 Research diary, F. Mkandawire, June 1998.
37 Research diaries, O. Munjanja, 26 September 1995, F. Mkandawire, March 1996.
38 Kanyama focus group, traditional educators, 13 September 1996, facilitator F. Mkandawire.
39 Research diary, F. Mkandawire, 8 May 1998; 10 May 1998.
40 Research diary, F. Mkandawire, 27 April 1998.
41 Research diary, F. Mkandawire, 27 April 1998; 6 May 1998.
42 Research diary, F. Mkandawire, 4 May 1998.

6 Target practice: gender and generational struggles in AIDS prevention work in Lushoto

Janet Bujra[1]

> *Teenage girls are susceptible to harrassment by men and boys, at the same time that they have to face punishment from older women*
> *(Tumbo-Masabo, 1994: 213)*

'Targeting' AIDS interventions towards social categories perceived to be at risk is often seen as the most efficient method of delivering health messages and changing behaviour. This chapter suggests that targeting may be problematic. First, it may justify the stigmatisation of categories already blamed for the spread of infection. Second, the exclusive focus on particular groups inhibits investigation of their relationships to others within a social setting (relations which can undermine or facilitate attempts to transform sexual behaviour and awareness).

Drawing on an example of AIDS prevention work in rural Tanzania, this chapter considers the way in which the epidemic has exposed and widened divisions between the generations. Focussing on interventions designed to protect young people from AIDS, it assesses the cross-cutting tensions between gender and generation in the context of discourse and action over safer sex, exploitation and power. Youth are not simply a 'social category' to be classified in terms of 'indices' of knowledge, rates of sexual activity, level of condom use etc. They must be seen in terms of their ambiguous place within the web of social relations. In this case, exploring the relations which older women and men (young and old) have with young women as the target for concern is crucial. Gender solidarity – even in the pursuit of HIV protection – cannot be assumed across the generations.

Response in Tanzania to the dangers facing youth in the context of AIDS has been two fold. There are the fears and concerns which the parental generation expresses for the safety of its children; there is also the fear of youth as a 'vector' of disease, lascivity and moral decline, often voiced by elders in general.

Parental concern is greatest at the point when normal sexual development puts young people at risk, not merely of overstepping the bounds of morality or of out-of-wedlock pregnancies (a long-standing and probably universal concern), but of fatal disease. This concern collides with a culturally sanctioned taboo on communication about sex between adjacent generations encountered in most areas of Tanzania (Van Eeuwijk and Mlangwa, 1997: 49; Tumbo-Masabo, 1998: 107; Baylies and Bujra *et al.*, 1999). In previous times sex education was generally dealt with through formal initiation for both young women and young men. Young people learnt about sexual propriety and pleasure in the context of general responsibilities to be shouldered by adults. Teaching was in the hands of the alternate generation of honorary grandparents with whom youngsters were allowed some licence. Where such institutions survive they are rarely in their original form (Ntukula, 1994; Katapa, 1998; Shuma and Liljestrom, 1998; Tumbo-Masabo, 1998). In response to the AIDS crisis, formal educational institutions have begun to face the need to educate young people about sex and sexual responsibility.

The prohibition on speaking of sexual matters between adjacent generations is bound up with a general distancing between parents and their children, summed up in the highly valued notion of 'respect' (*heshima*). To flout it is therefore to undermine broader parental interests. Conflicting emotions find confused expression: in the Lushoto area of this case study both men and women are shocked that, 'these days you can even refer to (sex) in front of your mother!' and they link this new freedom with children no longer respecting their parents. However, many parents now feel impelled to speak out: men to their children of both sexes, 'I will make the effort to tell them even though it is shameful'; even women to sons: 'We must tell (our sons) or we shall lose them'[2].

Whilst parents express terror at the dangerous prospects for their children, they have little confidence that their words of warning will be heard: as one mother said despairingly, 'Girls don't listen [to us]: our time is past'. This concern is not restricted to rural Lushoto (predominantly Muslim and patrilineal); it is echoed throughout Tanzania. In one of the capital city's peri-urban settlements (where wage employment and in-migration from many areas has produced a shifting and diverse population), women shared their anxieties in the very same words: 'when we speak to our sons about the dangers (of casual sex) they say 'your time is past'[3]. In Lindi, a rural Muslim but traditionally matrilineal community, an elderly man sums up 'the problem of youth' facing parents and society in general:

Today the boys and girls do not intend to live together in marriage. They look for relationships without permanence. They destroy their lives and catch various diseases. They need to be educated. Long ago they were better prepared for life than they are at present [through traditional initiation]. However, if todays's parents tell them about the past, their children say that all that has passed and that *they* live according to the current conditions of the world. 'You did as you did because you were not civilised'.

(quoted in Shuma and Liljestrom, 1998: 83)

If parents are fearful, elders in general are more condemnatory. In Lushoto they often portray young people as immoral and sexually promiscuous: 'Young people can't refuse (sex)', 'They have no shame'. Young women are 'more interested in making money [through selling sex]'. Worse than this, they are the source of disease: 'The young people especially bring [AIDS]', 'they just spread it'. The general view was that young women in particular run off to towns, become infected through casual sex or prostitution and return to die, taking others with them.[4] Sometimes elders blamed parents' lack of discipline for their daughters' sexual laxity. The contrast between the personal concern of parents and the general view of elders can be marked in Tanzania. In a study of one of the few facilities which support pregnant schoolgirls, Rugumyamheto (1998: 255) noted that local people 'found the idea of allowing unmarried girls who fell pregnant to continue with their education to be absurd and undesirable, whereas the parents of the girls appreciated the efforts'.

Parents have an interest in controlling youth and their sexuality. Young people still at home under parental discipline perform crucial labour tasks, especially girls who carry firewood and water, care for younger children and assist in cooking and cultivation. Unmarried men are also expected to be at parental bidding, though they enjoy more freedom and are able to evade demands. If young people marry those whom parents have chosen, then they link families and consolidate alliances between lineage groups. They bear children to further ancestral lines and enhance their parents' moral standing within the community. Young people who are out of control no longer provide labour; they shame parents with their flouting of rules and they may become a burden rather than a support. In Tanzania, when unmarried girls become pregnant, their chances of marriage (or at least of a creditable marriage) are severely limited. The fathers of their babies rarely marry them and grandparents (usually maternal) end up providing for the children.

Elders have an overall interest in young people acknowledging their authority and wisdom as custodians of customary practice. Ultimately this guarantees the perpetuation of the social order and ensures that people are supported in old age. This intergenerational 'bargain' has been put in question, not by AIDS *per se*, but by a history of social upheavals: the introduction of formal state education; the cash economy, urbanisation and the division of families through labour migration; and the political and economic incorporation of local communities (see Mbilinyi, 1979; Ishumi, 1984; Liljestrom *et al.*, 1998).

Intergenerational sex and AIDS

AIDS statistics in Tanzania reveal that the major group affected are young people, but also that the sexual relations through which it is transmitted are age-asymmetrical, with older men seeking younger women both for sex and marriage. Amongst women, those most heavily afflicted (AIDS cases) are women in the age category 20–29 whereas for men infection is heaviest amongst those aged 25–34 (NACP, 1998b: 14).

Older and more powerful men have always aimed to monopolise younger marriageable girls. In some areas the age differences are extreme: amongst the Wamwera, Shuma and Liljestrom (1998: 92) report a common pattern of men marrying women of their daughters' or even grand-daughters' generation. Intergenerational sex is given a deviant twist in the phenomenon of 'sugar daddies' (older men who exploit young girls for sex in exchange for soap, school fees or sodas). Some men are explicitly seeking 'safer' sex with girls they believe too young to be infected with AIDS.

Predating the AIDS epidemic is the noted reluctance of young men to marry, commented on in many studies (Rwebangira and Liljestrom, 1998; Mbilinyi and Kaihula, Chapter 4). With economic crisis and decline, young people of both sexes are hard hit. Pressures on peasant agriculture have led to an increasing influx of young people into towns without a concomitant rise in employment or other opportunities. Young women may resort to selling sexual services in order to survive, particularly if they fall pregnant and have children to support. Young men have no such option and marriage (for which they must provide bridewealth) is often beyond their immediate means. In the past it was customary for fathers, or maternal uncles, to contribute to such costs; nowadays these relatives are themselves pressed. It is cheaper for young men to pay for casual sex than to marry, especially if their partners are young women already supported by parents or a spouse (Katapa, 1998: 141). Moreover, young men may find themselves in competition with older and better-off men for the attentions of young women. Sexual networking cuts across generational boundaries.

In Lushoto, older village women were quick to censure older men, as well as parents, for the immoral behaviour of girls: 'We blame the men. It is men who seduce young girls'. The woman who said this then acted out a little play about how men do it – older men saying to young girls:

> 'let me show you something nice, you will like it'. No, no! 'Yes you will find it very nice. Come, I buy you soda, beer and roast meat'. And when the young girl is a bit drunk then it's all over with her! And maybe her parents think she is in school and she comes and says her head is hurting when it's something else altogether, but she can't say. Men are the destroyers of these young women.[5]

Although scenarios like this may go on in the village (where there was a bar selling sugar-cane beer), the elderly women were probably thinking of big cities or the nearby district capital (a frontier town of strangers) to which some young women gravitate, seeking work in bars and guest houses. However, structural inequalities also exist within the village and render young women the most vulnerable to unwanted sexual attention from men. The question is whether interventions designed to protect them from AIDS can be assured of support from older and more powerful people in the community, especially older women. Does gender solidarity in the interests of protection over-ride the tendency of the old to condemn the young for their sexual 'immorality', or even to see AIDS as an opportunity to reassert control?

AIDS: analysis and intervention in Tanzania

Generalised fears of young people's out-of-control sexuality may eventuate in moral panic demanding repressive measures. Campaigning interventions and the AIDS literature in Tanzania were initially dominated by a heavily moralistic focus on youth, but there has recently been a shift to more nuanced accounts acknowledging the dilemmas they face.

A major objective of NGO activity around AIDS in Tanzania has been in preventive work with youth. A listing of relevant NGOs (by no means exhaustive) was compiled in 1997 for the National AIDS Control Programme (Msaky and Kisesa, 1997). In Dar es Salaam it listed twenty-five organisations, more than one-third of which were focussed on youth, with only 12 per cent (three associations) concerned with gender issues. AIDS was first constructed as an issue of youth immorality, with interventions targeted at diverting young people from sexual activity. Organisations like UMATI (the Tanzanian Family Planning Association), WAZAZI (the Tanzanian Parents' Association) and EMAU (a Christian organisation aiming at better socialisation of young people) saw the issue at first as one of declining 'moral standards' amongst youth and were reluctant to promote knowledge, fearing that it would incite promiscuity (Van Eeuwijk and Mlangwa, 1997: 40).

A similar bias may be seen in the AIDS literature on Tanzania, excluding that employing a purely medical discourse. Of more than sixty publications reviewed for the period 1990–99, the largest category focusses on youth. In 1992, the World Bank recommended the Tanzanian government pay more attention to the risks facing young people. They also recommended the method: Information, Education and Communication programmes. 'Effective IEC has been recognised as the major tool available to combat the (AIDS) epidemic' (World Bank, 1992: 141). IEC programmes were based on the assumption that it was ignorance which fuelled risky sexual behaviour and spread AIDS. Globally this led to innumerable studies of 'knowledge, attitudes, beliefs and practice' (KABP studies) amongst given populations in order to assess their level of understanding. In Tanzania, as in other places, young people in schools constituted a captive population for monitoring. This choice of sample also coincided with a view of young people as the most vulnerable to HIV infection and the least under control.

Early KABP studies in Tanzanian schools often found a high level of AIDS awareness (e.g. Kapiga *et al.*, 1991; Klepp *et al.*, 1994; Ndeki *et al.*, 1994; Leshabari and Kaaya, 1997). However, they fuelled the anxiety of older people in confirming early sexual activity amongst young people, summarised here by Liljestrom *et al.* (1998: 29): 'Given the prevalence of the deadly HIV infection, it is alarming that more than 50 per cent of youth have had sexual intercourse by the age of 16'. Repressive responses amongst

researchers were initially common. Thus, Barongo *et al.* (1992) recommended: 'By-laws in each locality to prohibit or discourage premarital sex'
– though they also added 'and safeguard adolescents from promiscuous
adults'. Tibaijuka (1997: 52) advises: 'some combination of a conservative
abstinence upbringing campaign, and where necessary, early marriages after
the 18th birthday'. Teachers held similar views, with most refusing to teach
about condoms or to disclose where they might be obtained (Van Eeuwijk and
Mlangwa, 1997; Mgalla *et al.*, 1998). Indeed, Van Eeuwijk and Mlangwa
(1997: 49) question the title of 'knowledge' for what most young people are
told about sex: for them it is better described as 'rules and warnings'.

Over time, the positivistic assumptions of KABP-style studies have given
way to more qualitative approaches in youth research.[6] There is a shift in moral
perspective from repressive agendas towards more realism. A growing
acknowledgement of the dilemmas that face young people is evident; they
need to be taught negotiating skills as well as the value of condoms (see
especially Tumbo-Masabo and Liljestrom, 1994; Van Eeuwijk and Mlangwa,
1997). The premise that education can solve everything also undergoes a sea
change. Over-optimism and over-inflated claims, prominent in the KABP
studies, give way to a questioning of the 'assumption that inclusion of reproductive health issues in the curricula of primary and secondary schools will be
sufficient' (Kapiga, 1996: 441; Leshabari and Kaaya, 1997: 41). Youth
discourses, teaching methods and the language used to convey 'information'
are now held to be factors inhibiting straightforward 'knowledge-transfer'. The
receptivity of the audience is understood to be related to gender, age and the
prevalence of AIDS in the area (Nnko and Pool, 1997; Mgalla *et al.*, 1998).

There is another change. The cardboard cutouts, of 'promiscuous youth'
and of young girls as 'victims' of older males, give way to a more nuanced
view, with both boys and girls seen as pursuing complex strategies – the boys
to achieve free sexual access, the girls to gain material rewards through sex
without losing respect (Nnko and Pool, 1997; Leshabari and Kaaya, 1997).

In 1995–96, an AIDS curriculum was introduced into some of Tanzania's
primary schools. In some areas (e.g. Tanga) there was an active programme of
educational work, linking it with community action. The substance of the
curriculum was serious and accessible, though first-hand observation suggests
that there was little gender awareness in its promotion (e.g. girls and boys
were taught together) and denial regarding the actuality of young people's
sexual activities. That male teachers are sometimes found abusing young girls
is now acknowledged and addressed in some school programmes (Mgalla *et
al.*, 1998). UMATI has recently collaborated with the Swedish Association of
Sex Education (RFSU) to establish a peer education and advice service for
young people in which the distribution of contraceptives is reported to be an
accepted element (Fugelsang, 1997). However, 'pregnant schoolgirls' are still
expelled whilst their male partners continue their education (Puja and Kassimoto, 1994; Van Eeuwijk and Mlangwa, 1997; Mgalla *et al.*, 1998;
Ruguyamheto, 1998).

AIDS interventions with young people

If, amongst Tanzanian activists and researchers, there has been a growing recognition of young people's dilemmas in relation to AIDS, is this reflected in responses to young people in rural areas? Exploring the dynamics of women's organising efforts in rural areas, we sometimes found that gender solidarities were fractured by troubled inter-generational relations. One such social drama, unfolding over a period of 5 years, is described here. It raises two issues: how the targeting of groups at risk needs to encompass broader social relations and how easily AIDS interventions can be caught up in preexisting local conflicts and concerns.

In 1996, a girls' group was formed in the rural hinterland of Lushoto, a small district capital in the northern region of Tanga, Tanzania. A grouping of several hamlets scattered over mountains, the 'village' is populated by peasant farmers, predominantly Muslim and of a single ethnic group (Sambaa). Despite a long history of men (and more recently women) migrating to seek wage employment in plantations and urban centres, Lushoto district is not yet an area of high HIV prevalence.[7] The village (population approximately 3500) had one known AIDS death in 1996, two in 1997, three in 1998, none confirmed in 1999.

The local district hospital (one hour's walk away) has an AIDS Coordinating Officer and a Counsellor – it is also a testing and referral centre. AIDS interventions are mainly focussed on school students and on bar workers in the small towns in the district. Funding for AIDS work in the rural areas is scarce, though training for local midwives and healers has been forthcoming in some places. No such developments had occurred in the village under study.

Several AIDS initiatives were launched during the research period (1995–96). Following a baseline survey (1995)[8], which raised AIDS awareness, local people demanded 'seminars' (*seminaa*). Members of the research team in Tanzania (which included AIDS activists as well as scholars) organised a series of six community workshops. These were not passive didactic affairs but active, lively and participatory events. The method of *kuchokoza* (provoking) was used to stimulate local people to rethink the tragic situation of a disease spread through sexual relations, to break the silence and shame which had foreclosed open discussion and to plan personal and collective strategies to contain it. Single sex workshops were attended by men and women of all ages: in the end approximately 250 people took part. Each workshop chose two representatives – a younger and an older – to form a village group called 'The Coordinators' (six men and six women). This was to meet regularly to discuss AIDS issues in the village and to liaise with the local district hospital's AIDS Officer and AIDS counsellor, whom we had involved in the workshops.[9]

Investigation of an institution called *kidembwa* had also taken place. Middle-aged and elderly village women organise the collection of goods in cash and kind to support their members on the occasion of life crises (marriage, childbirth). Collections are accompanied by dancing and singing at the houses of members and (subversively in a Muslim community) the brewing and consumption of beer. These are women-only occasions from which men are excluded. *Kidembwa* is more like a network than a corporate group: membership is defined by continuing contribution and receipt of collections, drawing on different sets of women on each occasion depending on the location of the recipient's home and members' relation to her. There is no overall leadership in this activity, although there are acknowledged 'stars' in each small settlement making up the community.

These women perform a complex organisational task involving the disbursement of large amounts of money without the benefit of banks, paper or calculators (and which men deride as 'the money just goes round and round' – if they do not condemn it as sinful because of its link with alcohol consumption). The same women, by virtue of their age and energy and social knowledge, also play important roles as midwives and more generally in educating 'grandchildren' (their own and others) regarding sex and marriage (*wasomo*). Formal initiation ceremonies are beyond living memory in this area but there are informal arrangements which patchily cover the same ground: older women may police the transfer of a bride to her husband 'whole and pure' by inspecting the bedsheet on the wedding night, and by informing the bride beforehand what is about to happen to her and how she should respect her husband and his mother. Young people in trouble may confide in 'grandmothers' and obtain information about the facts of life. This generation of older women had promising organisational skills, capacities and social experience, which might have been productively harnessed to the fight against AIDS.

The girls' group (named Maisha or 'Life') was launched in response to a local woman leader's argument that young women were most vulnerable to HIV and least knowledgeable about it: a view confirmed by our baseline survey. In an area where there were no existing interventions I was pressed into this initiative as a key outsider. Our research project had adopted an ethical commitment to participation, but guarantees can never be given regarding the outcome of participatory work – it may well be problematic or have unintended consequences (Seeley *et al.*, 1992; Bond, 1997) whilst the researcher is inevitably caught up in competing political currents and pressures for validation.[10]

The plan was to initiate the group by recruiting the 1995–96 cohort of female school leavers from the local primary school and working with them to raise awareness of AIDS issues and provide forms of training or income generation which would offer an alternative to total and disempowering dependence on parents or their rebellious escape to towns seeking another life, with all its attendant risks. The idea was that these girls, none of whom had been chosen to go on to secondary education (there are limited secondary places for girls in this area), would, in the second year, initiate the succeeding cohort of school leavers, passing on to them the knowledge of HIV and how they could protect themselves. In this way membership of the group would roll over the years, with school leavers entering and older girls leaving as they became more confident and self-reliant – or moved away to marry (patrilocal marriage residence combined with exogamous patriclans meant that women married out, usually to other villages). In short, the intention behind the establishment of the girls' group was to further active learning of the dangers of AIDS and the risks of unprotected sex at the same time as providing a means to build young women's self esteem, capacity to stand on their own feet and to fight for their 'rights'.

The prospects for the girls' group looked particularly good as the woman leader, Ernestina, though younger than the major *kidembwa* leaders (she was 45 years old, whereas they were in their sixties or older), was a midwife and respected participant in *kidembwa* activities. Conversely, Ernestina had many characteristics that set her apart from others in the community. Although like other women she had married in patrilocally, she was not a Sambaa, but a Chagga, from Kilimanjaro. She and her husband were Christians, where the majority of Sambaa are Muslims (our survey uncovered only 12 per cent of Christians). Most local women have little education, but Ernestina had completed 8 years of primary school, trained as a nurse and worked independently for 5 years before her marriage. By 1995, she had lived in the village for more than 20 years. She had borne her husband eleven children and was fluent in the local vernacular. She told me she had 'become a Sambaa'.

Ernestina was also charming, warm, modest, untiring and full of ideas. As in the case of many strong women her husband was quiet and retiring, seemingly very proud of his wife's active work in the community. Her achievements were also promising. Whereas local women had little voice in political affairs, she had competed with her brother-in-law for the chairmanship of the hamlet in which she lived. Although losing this election she was chosen to become a women's representative on the village council (*halmashauri*). She organised a number of women's collective farming groups with aspirations to income generation. It was clear that there was some overlap between the personnel and activities of these groups and the instititution of *kidembwa*, suggesting that Ernestina had been building on existing foundations. During a meeting with Ernestina, members of one of these groups attended, mainly women with young children. Describing her relation to them, Ernestina explained that 'they call me 'mama''. In other words they were younger women than herself, and owed her a degree of respect.

In 1995 there was a political transition in Tanzania. The one-party 'socialist' system was being abandoned in favour of multi-party politics. Previously, all village political leaders had been representatives of the ruling party (*Chama cha Mapinduzi:* CCM); it was a condition of the job. Hence, Ernestina described herself as the representative of the UWT (*Umoja wa Wanawake wa Tanzania*) – the Party's women's wing. Now leaders were told not to make claims of political exclusiveness, although there were no village elections and the same leaders continued in office. A national election in 1996 saw the re-election of CCM. It then transpired that Ernestina had supported one of the opposition parties, unlike most people in the village whose loyalty to CCM remained unquestioning.

It was only gradually that the structural and ideological differences between Ernestina and others became apparent. Whilst there seemed at first to be no active male hostility towards her, men often dismissed her with a shrug, or a show was made of not remembering who she was. However, men would respond in the same contemptuous way when the *kidembwa* women were mentioned – *kidembwa* was a woman's affair, of no interest to them.

For almost a year the plan for the girls' group remained dormant as the harvest failed and times were hard. In 1996, Ernestina threw herself anew into the task. Within a few weeks she had located the primary school leavers of the previous year, and persuaded an elderly tailor to offer them lessons on a sewing machine. Approval was gained from the girls' parents by Ernestina and the tailor. In the next 2 months much was achieved. The group chose leaders and agreed to a name, the members each contributed a small amount so that an account could be opened in the bank in the district capital and Maisha was formally registered with the local office of the Ministry of Community Development. A grand celebration was planned to inaugurate the group and the girls threw themselves into preparations. Songs, dances and a play about AIDS were devised and rehearsed. The cycle of AIDS workshops was beginning and several of the girls attended one of the women's sessions. Parents, village political and religious leaders and some worthies from the district capital, even the local MP, were invited to the celebration. *Kidembwa* leaders called their followers to perform dancing and drumming in support.

The celebration was almost abandoned when three funerals of elderly men took place the same day – men to whom most people were related in one way or another and thus obligated to attend. *Kidembwa* women decided not to perform in deference to the funerals (heavily religious affairs). Although the MP did not arrive, and the audience of two or three hundred was mainly women and children, village political and religious leaders did attend, and speeches were given by the Village Chairman, a UWT leader from Lushoto town and Ernestina. The girls performed with panache and their efforts were greeted with loud and enthusiastic applause. One week later they repeated the performance for the girls in the higher classes of the village primary school.

Following this success, Ernestina and I approached the Village Chairman with a request for the allocation of some land for the group. The Chairman was pleased to oblige – he had at his disposal 'village land' which was no longer being cultivated collectively. Everyone was talking about the girls' group, and when the village AIDS Co-ordinators held their first meeting this was one of the groups that they decided to liaise with in the village (the others were the Village Council, the *kidembwa* network and young men's football teams).

With support and patronage from older women (both Ernestina and the *kidembwa* leaders) the Maisha initiative had to this point been an expression of cross-generational gender solidarity. It had also broken moulds. There is no tradition in this area of young women playing any public role. Following the completion of primary education, young women (*wasichana*) are expected to be silent and obedient, respectful towards parents and labouring at home and on their father's land until marriage. They are expected to remain innocent of men and of knowledge about sexual matters. In our baseline survey we had found such unmarried girls the most difficult to interview, often paralysed with embarrassment, sometimes literally turning away and covering their faces as we posed the questions. Initially they would deny knowing how AIDS was transmitted, though later answers betrayed more knowledge. Denial was culturally imposed through a discourse of 'shame'.

These appearances – of ignorance, shy reserve and compliance – were deceptive. Occasionally one met such girls in groups, returning from school or from collecting firewood and water. Collectively they were noisy and even daring. The 'moral panic' in the village about young women being out of control and running off to towns also suggested a different story. One of Ernestina's hopes was that the girls' group could divert young women from leaving. Although hers was the common assumption that girls who left did so in rebellion against parental authority and could only be heading for moral depravity, this should not be taken at face value. In areas of high population density like Lushoto where land is scarce, young people are often a drain on households. Young men have been migrating to towns for generations, look-ing for an independent income and the wherewithal to marry. They may stay away for years and never return to marry in the area. This leaves a prepon-derance of young women in rural areas whose chances of marriage are reduced. Many young people have relatives living away in urban areas, and extended visits to fathers, older brothers, uncles and aunts are common, during which some young people look for ways to stay on. It is not surprising that young women have begun to follow young men in these bids for inde-pendence. They do not necessarily end up in prostitution – they may find work as domestic servants or squeeze a living through petty trade, selling cooked food or sewing (Bujra, 2000b).

There was a pool of between twenty and thirty girls involved in the Maisha group at one time or another. Data was collected on twenty-three of these, through interaction, self-report, hearsay or follow-up interviews with a few of them 4 years later. In 1996, they were aged between 16 and 23 years, having completed the seventh and last year of primary education in the 2 preceding years. None had been chosen for secondary school. All were single, though at least two already had a child and two others were said to have been pregnant. They came from families across the village socio-economic spectrum, although this is narrow (most people are middle to poor peasant farmers with a better-off minority involved in trading and/or coffee growing). Of these twenty-three girls, nineteen were Muslims, four Christians. At least eight reported already having spent time away from the village, mainly visiting relatives in town, but at least two had experience of seeking and finding ways of earning an income (through domestic service and later selling cooked food in one case, through sewing in the other).

Their hopes and fears in joining Maisha were expressed in the following account by the young woman who had been chosen as 'secretary':

> In the meeting we were asked what we do once we have left school. We said that first we wait for the 'reply' [results of Standard 7 exams] and if we have failed we cultivate with our parents. We don't want to marry until we have become independent through learning skills. We agreed that fathers discuss things with their sons (but not with daughters). We could organise to buy cloth and sew it into clothes and sell them in the market…

They were over-optimistic about the opportunities for income generation projects and clearly saw the group in an instrumental way. These are what some of the young women said a few years later about their motivation to join:

> I thought I would get something.

> I joined for (self) development, for life.

> I wanted to learn sewing and other skills.

> I thought I would get a good life.

> (Interviews, 1999)

This optimism was tempered by their initial view of themselves as 'knowing nothing' and evidently having little faith in their ability to break the mould of established female lives. They did not question the gendered division of labour, which dictated for example that when land is cleared it is men who dig irrigation ditches; when bricks are made women bring water, but men mould the bricks. They expected to be married – though they were insistent that they would choose their own partners.

Despite the success of the sewing classes and the celebration, the difficulties of helping young women to organise themselves soon became apparent. Towards older women, particularly Ernestina, they adopted an attitude of excessive deference. Often the girls were silent, passive recipients of views, even when asked to offer their opinions. They were clearly used to being at the bottom of the social hierarchy, acted upon rather than acting. Conversely, Ernestina was used to being a leader, accustomed to taking the decisions and deserving shows of respect. She had little enthusiasm for democratic procedures or promoting the girls' autonomy and empowerment.

Contradictions soon began to emerge. The girls had courage to choose their own leaders only on an occasion when Ernestina was absent. She then sought to create a superior role for herself as *mlezi* of the group (an infantilising terminology– a *mlezi* is one who brings up or socialises children). The roles of 'chair', 'secretary' and 'treasurer' were new territory for the girls and as they said later: 'we didn't know what to do'. The need for formality of this kind was not only a matter of democratic accountability (my view) but also a condition for achieving recognition and possible 'help' (funding) from influential people outside the village – an objective to which Ernestina was clearly wedded. The Community Development Office in Lushoto town had a *mama maendeleo* (women's development officer) and donor funding was reputedly obtainable through them. This local agency of the state insisted on records of meetings before they would formally register the group. They also demanded a bank account; meanwhile the bank (at that point the only, state-owned, bank) would not accept the group's custom without the approval of the Community Development Office. We arranged a meeting with the *mama maendeleo* at which the girls were hectored on the importance of not having children too early! The Community Development officers offered no training in democratic procedures and no funds were forthcoming – a disempowering experience for the young women in the group.

Attempts to initiate the girls into the mysteries of keeping 'accounts' and the writing of 'minutes' were received by them without resistance, though their faces displayed expressions of fear and panic at the idea of shouldering such responsibilities. That they themselves might devise the constitution of the group was a startling idea – they expected Ernestina to lay down the rules and were happy for her to take on these awesome new responsibilities.

As the formal end of the research project approached, Ernestina pressed several ideas about further promotion of the group, eventually settling on a brick-making project. She had not involved the girls in discussion of these ideas. A source of external funding was discovered and I promised to help submit an application (it had to be in English), but only after meeting the group and ensuring their approval was gained. Again this was passive rather than active or questioning. Nineteen girls signed up to the application.

Soon afterwards the harvest again failed, and famine relief had to be supplied in the area. Maisha's attempt to plant together was abortive. The sewing lessons fizzled out, no meetings were called and the girls became disheartened. Several months later Ernestina's promotion of her plans, which had attracted attention in the district capital, bore fruit. A German NGO was looking for 'partners' in a project training women to build water tanks and Maisha was invited to participate. Even more unexpected was the news, received soon afterwards, that the funding application had been successful. If the celebration had put the young women of Maisha on the social map in the village, these developments were to lead to serious and prolonged dissension. There are several conflicting versions of the events, reflecting different social vantage points. These competing historical accounts were related and updated by the participants on succeeding brief visits made to the area in 1997, 1998 and 1999.

All agreed that the original Maisha group of young women had been replaced with a reconstituted group of older women; that young men had tried to get in on the funding benefits and failed; that gradually the collective welfare form of the project had been transformed into an entrepreneurial initiative. What few noticed was that the foundational impetus of the whole enterprise – to address the AIDS epidemic – had largely been forgotten. An account of the different versions of history may begin with that of original members of Maisha, six of whom were interviewed in 1999.

Competing accounts of history: the Maisha girls

Only one of the original members was still active in the new Maisha group – her position will be considered separately. The others saw themselves as having been abandoned: Ernestina 'left us and went off after those older women'. Their places were taken by, as one put it, 'those *kidembwa* women' or as another termed them, 'big people'. 'They stole our group'. Two of them admitted that by the time the brick-making money came through they had gone away to towns, though one (the original Chair) had asked that she still be counted in. All said they were still keen and had not lost interest, but there were no meetings, no sewing lessons, no more teaching about AIDS. One said that Ernestina had 'stopped coming and left us to manage on our own', whilst another admitted that Ernestina was herself discouraged as girls dropped out. One said that some girls 'got married and moved away', whilst another suggested that 'husbands don't like their wives to go out'. When the brick-making funds arrived they assumed that they would be called, but they were not. Rumours began to spread. 'People said that Ernestina was eating the money and we were not sure. We thought you had sent the money and she had taken it'.

The girls conceded that they had done little to challenge these developments. They did not get together as a group, though they talked bitterly to each other when they met. Two of the girls wrote to Ernestina, in collaboration with two young men [see below], asking her to come and talk to them, 'but she did not come'. They did not see how they could confront Ernestina: 'she is too big and she knows [best]'. 'We thought you would come back and we said "let's wait" '. 'We were afraid of her'. 'We were oppressed and we didn't do anything. We were divided'. 'We didn't see any solution so we just left it'. 'Please don't tell her we have said these things'. They now realised the value of accountability – of calling meetings, of discussing the accounts. 'Since you went we have never been to the bank'. 'We don't know what happened to the money in the bank'.

This passivity did not mean that the girls had not appreciated the group. They valued even the sewing lessons, albeit with only one machine and limited materials. The celebration, which thrust socially invisible young women onto the public stage, had a particular thrilling impact on them. One remembered her role with pride: 'I led the dancers! I was the one with the hat!'. This had been a high point when the group coalesced; it had also been an effective mode of active learning about AIDS. The play, which the girls and Ernestina devised, took up a theme about living positively with AIDS which was reiterated in the workshops. A young woman goes to town and comes home infected, and at first she is avoided out of fear. Then her friends rally round, insisting that AIDS is not contracted through everyday social contact and should not be seen as a shameful secret. The young woman is supported to live (though the events which led to her infection are not confronted!). This simple story enacted by them spoke more effectively than some of the other 'information' relayed in the workshops. As one young woman said of that 4 years later: 'I have forgotten it all now'.

More than one villager commented that the workshops had broken the public silence about AIDS. A mother of one of the Maisha girls went further:

> Our daughters began to ask, 'Mama what is AIDS?' and although we don't talk with our children about these things we began to explain to them how dangerous it is these days to have sex with someone. This was because of Maisha. They didn't know these things.

The members' sense of the dangers facing young women had been heightened – the risks of unprotected sex, of multiple partnerships and of their vulnerability to sexual coercion. However, their sense of empowerment in relation to these dangers had hardly been enhanced. None of the six who were interviewed 4 years later had ever negotiated the use of condoms in sexual encounters even whilst they nearly all thought that condoms should be available to young people. Two had been raped: one in the village – in consequence of which she became pregnant and is now considered unmarriagable,[11] the other in Mombasa, where she had worked as a domestic servant. A third had experienced a 'marriage by capture' – a suitor had come and carried her off without the usual formalities. She connived in this at first, and her parents accepted the union, but she was then repelled by the man's forceful sexuality. He was a trader, often away in Dar es Salaam where she believed he had many other partners. She was now afraid of him: 'he may infect me'. The positive outcome was that she had returned to her parents and was seeking a divorce.

Four of the six young women were now married, three to men who were involved in urban trading (i.e. a risky situation for wives left at home). Even if they were happy with their partners, they knew that a wife could not refuse sex, even if she had suspicions. 'You are a wife, what can you do?' Men were seen as sexually voracious by nature: 'They are made like that and you can't do anything'. They also pointed out that a young wife who refuses sex will be subject to public criticism from the same elderly women who divulge the secrets of sex to them on marriage (*wasomo*): 'If you refuse sex he may send for your *msomo* and she will be angry: "you will shame us. You are married, you have to do it" '.

Other versions of events

Ernestina's account of events was very different to that of the girls. She argued that when the funds and the invitation to construct tanks came through, the Maisha girls had already lost interest in the group. Many had married and gone to join husbands too far away to continue their involvement (in 1997 she named twelve out of my sample of twenty-three who were now married). The funding opportunity was too good to miss, however, so she resurrected 'Maisha' with women who were mainly from her previous 'UWT' groups – married women with young children. One of these women said later: 'Mama Ernestina came to ask me to join, saying that she could depend more on older women who would stay put'. Ernestina claimed she had contacted the previous members, offering to return the entrance fee to those who did not wish to continue (a claim they flatly denied). Only one of the original members had rejoined – Ernestina claiming this as evidence that the original Maisha had not died. This young woman had more need of the group than any other member – she was the girl who had been raped and was bringing up her child with the help of her parents. Marriage was not an alternative mode of survival for her.

As far as external donors were concerned, the original Maisha group, with its original aims (amongst which AIDS awareness training for young women was paramount and income generation a means to that end) was the recipient of funding. The new group, however, was focussed far more narrowly on creating a business. In these terms, the brick-making project was a great success, with Ernestina's energy and organising capabilities ensuring that the women learnt new skills and produced thousands of cement bricks. However, these were too expensive for village people and it was not long before the brick-making machines were relocated to the district capital and the women went every day to work there. Four years later the work groups had dwindled. Then Ernestina became sick for a while, and without her sales efforts, orders declined.

Democratic procedures and practice were no more a feature of the new group than of the old. There was considerable doubt that profits had been divided fairly, and no-one ever went to the bank except Ernestina, nor were regular meetings held. Planning decisions were generally taken by Ernestina herself. Given the success of Maisha in attracting external funding, she had encouraged several of the elderly *kidembwa* women to copy it – to form a group (tellingly called 'Hope') and to contribute money to open a bank account. They claimed that: 'It was Ernestina who took the money to the bank' and they had seen no evidence of the account having been opened. Neither the new members of Maisha nor the elderly *kidembwa* women had been able to challenge Ernestina, despite corrosive suspicions. Leaders were not people to be questioned – you simply followed, accepting that they knew best. 'We don't like to be seen as difficult people' said two women in the new

Maisha group. By this stage then, relations between Ernestina and other older women had lost their positive edge.

The other versions of these events cast more light on gender relations. Village men could not accept that the funding was for women alone. They saw the donation (and later the equipment which was purchased with it) as belonging to the village as a whole. They set up Ernestina as the villain of the piece, but also blamed women in general for not confronting her: 'The problem with women in this place is that they are fearful creatures'. They did not offer male support, though 4 years later the co-ordinators' group was rehearsing plans to intervene.

A sub-theme was the particular hostility of young men. Initially, they were jealous of the girls' success and some of them planned a parallel group focussed on football teams. Later they were encouraged by Ernestina into thinking they might share in Maisha's fortune. Some of them joined the girls in cultivating their plot, digging ditches and clearing the ground. After the harvest failed they were marshalled by her to fetch and carry heavy loads and move the brick-making machines; but when the machines were removed to the district capital they found themselves excluded from the action like the young women. This led to a brief alliance of the disaffected across gender lines (the letter sent to Ernestina), but it was fuelled merely by anger and came to nothing. In the same way that older women responded to the girls' newfound solidarity with increasing attempts at control, older men derided the young men's efforts: 'They were too impatient. They wanted to eat too quickly'. It is notable that Ernestina had exploited the young men to carry out stereotypically male jobs.

Conclusions

Two questions have been addressed here. The first is why campaigning interventions and the AIDS literature in Tanzania came to be dominated by a focus on youth and a heavily moralistic agenda. The second is why a project in rural Tanzania in which building bridges between the generations was a key feature, nevertheless fell short of its goals. Linking these two questions is the argument that generational relations, like those of gender, have become more charged in the era of AIDS as youth are seen as a dangerous vector of disease and a threat to the moral order. A common response has been attempts to reassert the control of the older over the younger generation through measures of repression. The project described here aimed at different objectives, but it was subverted to the same ends. The notion of independent young women controlling their own affairs and devising their own responses to sexual coercion proved too revolutionary for an older generation who preferred, by omission or commission, to remind them of their dependence. In this endeavour they were successful, because they were able to build on young women's structural weakness and on their unquestioning habits of respect for elders. That young women 'marry out' also created difficulties in stabilising a group based on locality. The very success (in material terms) of the project led older women to appropriate its benefits for themselves and to sideline the young people for whom it had originally been devised.

This complex and contested unfolding of what began as an intervention around AIDS can be interpreted through more than one lens. Though personalities were clearly at issue, so too were structural tensions. Many local people explained the outcomes abstractly as 'bad leadership' (*uongozi mbaya*). However, in this setting there is no clear model for more democratic, inclusive or accountable forms of leadership amongst women – though some of the formalities of village government under 'socialist democracy' might have been asserted. Of course women are largely excluded (and to some extent exclude themselves) from positions of political leadership in the village. The institution of *kidembwa* is inclusive in its way for the generation of older women, but its leaders derive their authority from trust and respect for elders, rather than from formal procedures of election and accountability.

There is also some truth in what men say here: that women are fearful of speaking out, of challenging authority, or demanding their rights.[12] This is most evident amongst unmarried girls, but it is also true of older women. Such older women find themselves in an ambiguous position. As mothers or as elders in the *kidembwa* they are dedicated to policing marriage and sexuality, ultimately to the benefit of men as husbands. Whilst the institution of *kidembwa* has some subversive aspects, these are submerged and hidden. Secret beer drinking may cement female solidarity but any dialogue or challenging of male prerogatives is avoided. At the same time, it is evident that older women could use their position vis à vis younger women to support and protect them more. Young women are eager and ready to respond to initiatives from older women and it is to their grandmothers that they turn as mediators in case of serious problems (rape, fear of infection). In the case of Maisha, the promise of cross-generational support was not sustained. The *kidembwa* leaders were unable to confront Ernestina even on their own account, and did not do so on behalf of the young women of Maisha. I have cited another telling instance elsewhere (Bujra and Baylies, 1999: 42). In one of the women's workshops when a young woman asked daringly, 'Aren't there any condoms for women?', an elderly *kidembwa* woman turned and glared at her: 'Who said that? You young women are too much! You want it (sex) too badly... People will say you are a prostitute!'

As an AIDS initiative, the Maisha project had some success at the level of discourse and understanding as well as tentative organisational initiatives, but it got entangled in gendered and generational tensions. It was also subverted via the temptations for personal advancement offered by external funding, thus underlining a general dilemma in AIDS work – that the urgency of immediate needs outweighs long term strategies for survival. Designing AIDS interventions that offer support to those (women, youth) who challenge existing power structures is crucial. It is also clear that the work will not bear fruit if it is targeted on a single social category, since it is the *relations between such categories* that are the source of constraints and tensions, whilst they also offer possibilities for creative work.

Notes

1   Acknowledgement of the contribution of many others to the Lushoto project is due, especially Haji Ayoub and Helena Anthony, research assistants, but also Naomi Kaihula and Julius Mwabuki who facilitated workshops in the village in 1996. Nothing could have been achieved or learnt without the co-operation, support and enthusiastic participation of people in the village, to whom I express my gratitude. To respect confidentiality and preserve anonymity I have not named the village and all names are pseudonyms.
2   Quotations from baseline survey, 1995.
3   Feddy Mwanga, fieldnotes, Tegeta, 1995.
4   Quotations from baseline survey and interviews with village leaders, 1995.
5   Group discussion with *kidembwa* leaders, 1995.
6   The value of survey techniques and sophisticated statistical calculations is in doubt in the field of sexuality (see methodological Appendix, Chapter 2). A combination of qualitative and quantitative techniques is more productive in this field, if each is sensitively and appropriately employed.
7   Personal communication from Lushoto district Hospital indicated a 6.8 per cent HIV prevalence rate amongst blood donors in 1998 (most blood donors are males); compared with a national prevalence of 7.6 per cent for men and 11.6 per cent for women (NACP, 1998b: 6).
8   The survey, delivered in Swahili or Kisambaa, covered a structured sample of one hundred respondents, fifty men and fifty women, with quotas for people of different socio-economic levels and ages. (See Chapter 2). Haji Ayoub accompanied me in interviewing men, Helena Anthony in interviewing women. Questions ranged widely around views of AIDS and what might be done about it.
9   Some of the deliberations of this group have been described elsewhere (Bujra and Baylies, 1999; Bujra, 2000a) and an excerpt from their first discussion is quoted in Chapter 9.
10   A particular issue emerged when anticipations were foisted upon me, based on local people's experiences of 'outsiders' and 'development projects'. Whereas my view was that initiatives should be defined by and under the control of local people (although which local people is problematic), they tended to see such developments as dependent on all-powerful 'donors' (*wafadhili*), who at best may be co-opted. My aim was to support the initiatives of others, with the intention not to organise, but to observe the way in which people organise themselves. Whilst I made some small material inputs as a gesture of support, I offered no major financial contribution. Some participants found this both confusing and disappointing; conversely they tended to assume that the funding for the brick-making project came from me. Other issues arose as the project developed, with a difference of views between myself and Ernestina in relation to democratic procedures and to bids for, and the use of, external funding.
11   The young man was brought before a village court but only forced to pay the expenses of delivery in recompense for his crime.
12   The contrast with Rungwe women is marked (see Chapter 4)

7 Reconciling individual costs with collective benefits: women organising against AIDS in Mansa

Carolyn Baylies

This chapter considers the factors that make community-based interventions around HIV/AIDS successful – what works, why and for whom? If gender relations are fundamental to the transmission of AIDS, the way collective activity addresses and impacts on them is critical. In this regard, the answer to the question, 'what works', applies not just to the sustainability of an initiative, but its capacity to confront gendered power in getting to the heart of the epidemic.

With reference to Mansa in Luapula Province, the activities of several groups will be discussed.[1] Consideration will be given to the way in which collective interventions around AIDS can make productive use of organising capabilities so as, first, to meet immediate objectives of providing care or increasing AIDS awareness and, second, to have 'spillover' effects on the lives of participants, through increasing their ability to protect themselves and their families against HIV. In the process, the question of how the personal costs and benefits of engaging in collective action around AIDS are calculated and reconciled by participants will be addressed. How are individual costs in time and foregone income, for example, balanced against a collective benefit of greater awareness and more protective behaviour? Is it essential to link issues of economic compensation or economic security to AIDS activities? What kind of external support can benefit such initiatives and at what point in their development?

Before considering these issues, the logic behind support for community-based initiatives and for strategies highlighting women's role in respect of them can be sketched out more fully. As Parker (1996) notes, AIDS work has increasingly shifted from an emphasis on individuals, towards strategies designed to 'equip vulnerable communities more adequately with the tools necessary to address their own vulnerability' (1996, S29). This emphasis resonates with more general support for participation in the development process as a means towards achieving greater democracy and fuller realisation of the capabilities of community members. A participatory, bottom-up approach acknowledges the legitimacy of local knowledge and the ability of individuals to know and verbalise their needs (Bond and Vincent, 1997). It also assumes that those who have been disadvantaged in the past can increase their chances of securing justice and greater equality through collectively promoting an agenda expressing their needs (Oakley *et al.*, 1991; Burkey, 1993). What is emphasised is not just the locating of projects or initiatives in groups, but activity which, in forging cohesion, challenges those structures which create or perpetuate inequalities. The group, from this perspective, has a dynamic which can impact on individuals, strengthening them in their individual capacity (Rowlands, 1997).

Such approaches can sometimes regard the disadvantaged as more homogeneous than they actually are and neglect the way in which participation can be hierarchical in nature, as can the benefits it confers. Collective activity, which takes little account of gender differences, for example, can perpetuate existing gendered power relations. If collective action of those politically and economically disadvantaged is an expression of their resistance and agency in general terms, however, then collective activity of women may similarly serve to counter disadvantage specifically defined by gendered power relations. Thus, Sen and Grown (1988: 89) see women's organisations as central to strategies for empowerment, arguing that for women to move beyond their current situation, they need not just 'to strengthen their organisational capacity', but also to 'crystallise visions and perspectives'.[2]

Women's groups and the utilisation of women's informal networks have featured in the literature on interventions around AIDS (McNamara, 1991; Heise and Elias, 1995; Reid, 1997). As noted in Chapter 1, Ulin (1992: 67) has encouraged an exploration of links between women's networking capacities, personal empowerment and behavioural change and has argued that women's informal associations may be a 'powerful vehicle for normative change'. Du Guerny and Sjöberg (1993: 1029) affirm that women's facility for organising self-help groups can be an important resource in AIDS work, which can also 'strengthen and empower women'.

The extension of women's networks into new areas, and the utilisation of their organisational capacities in new ways, can challenge the *status quo* of gendered social spaces. This is particularly important with HIV/AIDS, where linkages between vulnerability and means of prevention need to be revealed, if the structural factors which can impede safe practices are to be addressed. There is strategic value, therefore, in beginning with those most vulnerable, capitalising on their strengths, and moving outward to encompass those with whom their vulnerability is constructed. For if otherwise, relations of vulnerability may simply be reproduced and remain unchallenged. If women assert the need for community level responsibility and protection, moreover, through taking matters outside of the household and beyond the couple, this may of itself force reconsideration of gendered spheres of responsibility. That such initiatives are women-led and women-defined – at least in the first instance – may be important in contributing to a reversal of women's subordination in other respects.

The following account, which examines collective action around AIDS in Mansa, is based on research carried out between 1995 and 1999. Following an initial review of AIDS activities in the area, a base-line survey was conducted in early 1996 in Chitamba, on the outskirts of Mansa. In April and May of that same year a series of focus group discussions were held among men and women in different age categories. From May 1996, the activities of a number of groups involved directly or indirectly with AIDS activities were monitored. Periods of more intensive observation and follow-up occurred in July and August 1996, December 1996, July 1998 and August 1999, during which meetings were attended, individual interviews were conducted and a series of group discussions held.[3]

The setting

Mansa is the provincial headquarters of Zambia's Luapula Province, in the northern part of the country. The town has a population of some 50,000, and is a bustling commercial centre through which traders pass bringing fish from Lake Mweru and the Luapula river to the north, and Lake Bangweulu to the east, on their way to Zambia's Copperbelt. It is characterised by a moderately high level of HIV prevalence and, as in many towns in Zambia, the presence of the epidemic intrudes with uncomfortable immediacy. Those with whom we worked were themselves affected, often having to break off their work to attend funerals. The research period saw the death of a local UN volunteer who co-ordinated the AIDS youth programme in the town, school teachers, the founder of one of the groups we observed, and the husbands of several members of another. Their illnesses were not always diagnosed. There was limited voluntary or even clinical testing occurring, primarily because of a disinclination of many to verify their HIV status, but also because of the sporadic supplies of reagents.

Despite uncertainty, however, people knew this illness and lived with it on a day to day basis. Of those in our base-line survey in Chitamba, 79 per cent said they had known someone with AIDS and 80 per cent considered it to be a problem within the local community. In 1994, an estimated 23 per cent of pregnant women in Mansa were infected with HIV (Fylkesnes, 1995).[4] Subsequent estimates for adult prevalence put the figure variously at 21 and 29 per cent, translating into an estimated 4,300 to 6,000 adults in the town living with HIV or AIDS (UNAIDS/WHO 2000b; Ministry of Health, Zambia, 1997).

As in other locales, a greater proportion of women (72 per cent) than men (56 per cent) considered themselves to be in personal danger from HIV.[5] Although views were neither uniform nor static, many women considered that prevailing cultural norms permitted them little means of protecting themselves, particularly within marriage. The common refrain: 'women are faithful but men are a problem' was reiterated here.[6] However, specific repercussions of AIDS also coalesced around the situation of widows in relation to the practices of property grabbing and sexual cleansing. Among the members of a small widows' association formed in the mid 1990s in Mansa to seek means of mutual support, for example, only one had avoided having property held jointly with her husband being seized by her in-laws on his death.[7] If this is a particularly graphic example of rights being abused, cleansing of a widow is a more symbolic expression of subordination. This may take different forms, but when entailing sexual intercourse between a widow and a male relative of her late husband, it can be a highly dangerous practice for both partners.[8]

Research in Mansa centred on the catchment area of the Buntungwa Health Clinic, one section of which was a suburb on the northern edge of the town, which featured a school, several churches, and the Muchinka market among its blocks of council houses. The other, separated from the suburb by a stream, comprised a cluster of villages known collectively as Chitamba, where there were a number of shops and, at the far end, another primary school. Scattered among the mud brick houses were many whose residents sold local beer or small amounts of produce. It was in Chitamba that our base-line survey was carried out. Members of focus groups were drawn both from there and from the neighbouring suburb, as were the groups whose progress we charted.

Chitamba was founded as a village in the 1950s when a Catholic priest travelled with members of his former congregation from a place called Chitamba in Northern Province (hence the name) and settled near the Mansa river. These Bemba settlers were joined by people from the locality[9] and later by retired civil servants who wished to remain in the vicinity but no longer had claim to government housing and, as government housing itself became increasingly scarce, by others in need of local accommodation. The population of the area was relatively mobile, many having spent periods of their life (often during their schooling) in other parts of the province, on the Copperbelt or elsewhere in Zambia. Only 13 per cent of those surveyed said they were born locally.

Some of those in Chitamba farmed, but their land was often as far as 10 kilometres away. Some were in wage employment and some in trade.[10] As both a district and provincial headquarters, with a hospital, two urban health centres and a number of schools and training centres, Mansa town had a core of salaried individuals. However, there were also high levels of poverty, exacerbated by redundancies following the closure of its only factory, privatisation of parastatal organisations and the reduction in the size of some government departments. In Mansa district as a whole, 48 per cent of households were classified as 'core poor', 18 per cent as 'poor' and only 34 per cent as 'non-poor' in the mid 1990s (Seketeni *et al.*, 1995).[11]

The connection between economic difficulties and the spread of HIV was not lost on the local population. One member of a group of civil servants observed that 'the figures of those unemployed are shooting up because the government has put in place structural adjustment'. He considered the ensuing hardship to households to bear most heavily on young women: 'those who can't find work resort to prostitution'.[12] In consequence, attention to economic problems and a focus on generating income for communities, households and particularly women figured prominently in programmes on AIDS in the area.

AIDS activities in Mansa

Mansa enjoyed a fairly high level of intervention around AIDS from early in the epidemic. Its more recent experience provides a glimpse of attempts to devolve AIDS work to health centres and local communities. This reveals modest accomplishments, but also frustrations. A pattern in Mansa and elsewhere in the province has been that initiatives begin with enthusiasm on all sides, and then slip away because of bureaucratic problems, lack of sustained support and misunderstandings about the balance between community service and individual compensation.

Churches have been active in AIDS work elsewhere in the province, assisted in part through external support.[13] However, in Mansa their involvement has been limited.[14] Much more important have been initiatives carried out within the government sector, especially at district level, bolstered and supplemented by a programme of UNDP sponsored assistance.[15]

In the early 1990s, for example, UNDP helped to set up the Muchinka Teen Centre in conjunction with the local council and supported by funding from UNICEF (Raja, 1993). Recognising that lack of economic opportunities and restriction of recreational facilities could conspire to place young people in unsafe situations, the intention was to provide a place for sports, drama and AIDS education. In association with this centre, and progressed by a series of international and local UN volunteers, a tailoring project to train young women and a street kids project to provide income generation for out of school youth were set up. A counselling and home-based care programme was also put in place, and in 1993 UNDP assisted as the district embarked on programmes of devolving AIDS activities to the locality. This involved training both 'psycho-social counsellors', who were to work out of health centres, and twenty to twenty-five community-based counsellors in each of the catchment areas serviced by these centres.

Various of these initiatives encountered problems of sustainability. After initial enthusiasm over the Muchinka Teen Centre, for example, lack of incentives prompted six of the fourteen volunteer trainers in drama or sport to drop out within the first 4 months.[16] While one of those trained as community-based counsellors in Chitamba was conducting AIDS education on an individual basis in 1995, there was little evidence of other activity, and when a refresher course was held in 1995, less than half attended. One of those originally trained explained that when the programme began, we 'were even given transport to reach out to the villages. After some time, people started withdrawing. Some wanted to be paid something. Others were quarrelling amongst themselves as to who was to use the bicycles'.[17]

Mansa was not unique in this regard. In other parts of the province, attempts to generate community-based AIDS activities met with a similar fate. In Kawambwa district, where ninety people were trained as community carers, few remained active, partly because of lack of transport but also, according to the district AIDS co-ordinator, because they 'were not happy about being volunteers; they would have liked to have had a small allowance'.[18] That this reflects a general problem is indicated by the conclusion in a review of Zambia's AIDS programme conducted in 1997, that 'the lack of incentives, including the lack of a means of identity and/or encouragement, undermines both HBC (home-based care) and IEC (information, education and communication) programmes, especially at grass roots level' (Republic of Zambia, 1997: 4).

Efforts both to continue fostering community service and to address the issue of poverty have converged in a strategy to combine AIDS work at community level with income generation. Calling on people at community level – and especially women – to come together in income generating projects has been a theme in Zambia for some time, if sometimes pursued in a rather unreflective fashion, eliciting in turn a mechanistic response (Harrison, 1997). In the context of AIDS, however, it is given particular urgency and deeper meaning by the conviction in some quarters that women need to gain greater financial autonomy if they are to be successful in protecting themselves against HIV. This was reflected in the comment of the provincial IEC specialist in Luapula, for example that 'the best thing to do first is to empower the women economically and everything else will fall into place'.[19]

A shift towards the promotion of income generation as part of an AIDS strategy occurred in Mansa District in the mid 1990s. Refresher courses set up for community-based counsellors proved to be an 'eye opener' to district and provincial staff, given the expressions of discontent and recriminations over lack of support emerging from participants. (Maarugu, 1995: 8). It became clear that while personal poverty undermined the motivation of individual counsellors, the poverty of the community meant that there were few means of meeting the needs of affected families, even for such basics as soap and food. In consequence, 'initiation of community based income generating projects was recommended as the only panacea to the prevailing irksome problem' (Maarugu, 1995: 8,9). The provincial permanent secretary stamped official approval of this strategy, particularly in respect of a focus on women, in his remarks in Mansa on World AIDS Day in December 1996:

> From now on we want to witness the springing up of women's income generating groups... managed by these groups with technical and financial support of the social welfare department and other interested donor agencies. It is my hope that through taking such activity oriented approaches that we will be practical in the fight against HIV and in taking care of the AIDS patient we may tackle some of the root causes of the infection.[20]

Collective activity around AIDS in Mansa

In order to examine more closely the factors which contribute to or undermine the effectiveness of community-based AIDS work in Luapula, we focus on three groups in Mansa, concentrating on one, the Muchinka Women's Drama Group and using the other two, the Natweshe Development Club and Lisach as examples of contrasting experience. The three groups differ in terms of the relation between income generation and AIDS work and accordingly in the specifics of their histories. The Women's Drama Group was formed expressly to do AIDS work. It added income generation as a means for sustaining this primary activity and providing some individual benefit. The Natweshe Club was originally formed for the specific purpose of income generation, but then added AIDS activities to its overall set of objectives. The Lisach group was formed to foster greater self reliance and economic autonomy among widows and families affected by AIDS and combined health education, skills training and income generation from the beginning. Drawing upon their respective fortunes, some insight may be gained concerning the sustainability of AIDS initiatives with respect not just to what works, but what works for whom and in what way.

The Muchinka Women's Drama Group

Eight women who regularly traded in the enclosed market in Muchinka, not far from Butungwa Clinic, came together in April 1996 to form a drama group in order to raise awareness about the dangers of AIDS. This was partly inspired by a focus group organised by the research team, in which five of the women had participated, and which had galvanised their individual concerns about AIDS. However, it also drew on the vision and previous experience of one of the women, who had participated in a similar group in the heart of the fishing area in the north of the province. Most of the women belonged to the United Church of Zambia and had been active in its women's group, but some belonged to other churches. All had children and, save for one who was widowed, all were married. Most had been educated no higher than the primary level. Their average age was 34 years.[21]

Within a short time they had worked up a play to performance level. They were eager not just to use drama to teach other women how HIV/AIDS could be prevented, but also to help orphans and assist in the care of AIDS patients in the community. However, they were quite clear that to do so required support and resources. Based on her earlier experience, their leader asked the research team to provide allowances for their performances. They pointed out that they were sacrificing their time which would otherwise be spent at the market, earning money for their families. How could they do this extra work without some compensation?[22] Since their determination to form the club had been sparked by the focus group – had we not asked what they themselves could do about AIDS? – it was perhaps not unreasonable that they would turn to the research team for assistance. This issue rumbled for some time, through discussion about personal costs and about who were the immediate and ultimate beneficiaries of their drama, and whether it made more sense for them to claim allowances (and if so, from whom?) or to support their activities through some collective income generating activity.[23]

In August 1996, they performed a series of plays at the Buntungwa clinic. One, 'The wandering husband', generated animated and frank discussion, which moved from an observation that the play 'was teaching how women could be unfortunate due to circumstances beyond their control' to the assertion that 'women should demand that men use condoms' to the plea that 'men should also be sensitised'.[24] A key moment for the group occurred towards the end of that month when they were invited to perform for a group of UNDP officials from Lusaka. The visitors were greatly impressed and encouraged the women to submit formal proposals to their local colleagues for further assistance.[25] However, the group was unhappy about the paper trails they were being asked to initiate: 'we don't talk in papers. Papers do not speak'. They wanted a face to face discussion.[26] And though wary lest government officials take credit for their initiative (when 'this could not be credited to anyone but us'[27]), they were assisted in registering as a group by the provincial IEC specialist who also sought funding on their behalf. This eventually bore fruit and towards the end of 1996 the group received a grant from UNDP, which they used to purchase commodities for sale in the market, a portion of the profit going to support the group's activities.[28]

One year later, at the end of 1997, the Muchinka drama club was invited by local UNDP workers for training in peer education and writing action plans (the fashion of the day). It was hoped that skills acquired would be put to use in community work. In the event it was only the drama club, among several groups attending the workshop, which took up further activities, mostly associated with providing care and comfort for AIDS patients.[29] Around this time they also received another grant via the UNDP, this time in the form of one hundred chicks and chicken feed in accord with their request to be supported in a poultry project. Throughout the following months, they performed on a number of occasions, including World Health Day, 7 April 1998, when the Permanent Secretary for the province donated a small amount to them in recognition of the contribution they were making to the community.[30] A performance for Zambia's resident UNDP representative yielded a further donation of a number of bags of mealie meal, which they subsequently distributed in connection with their home care work. They also received a grant from the government's 'constituency development fund'.[31]

In the spring of 1998, they auditioned for a representative of the Society for Family Health, the body distributing Maximum condoms, which was looking for a drama group to educate the community on the importance of using condoms. Having been selected, a contract was signed on their behalf by the District Medical Office, according to which they were to perform 3 days a week, receiving K15,000 (equivalent to about $8) per performance.

In preparation they received additional training as community-based contraception educators. The contract lasted for some 6 months, and though they were unhappy about its terms, feeling that they were not fully compensated for their time and costs incurred, it allowed them to branch out and gain additional standing within the community.

By September 1999, they had completed their contract with the Maximum distributors and were contemplating future directions. The poultry project begun in early 1998 had been moderately successful, but had depended on the use of the chicken run of one of the members who subsequently wished to use it for her own purposes. Having therefore decided to build their own chicken run, the group needed funds to buy chicks and feed and were considering using some of their banked savings for this purpose. Drawing on their marketing skills and a certain capitalist canniness, they considered purchasing beans or groundnuts and holding them until the price rose in order to make a profit. If they could buy the chicks on the basis of this speculative enterprise, they thought they could then approach a potential funder for the rest.

Members of the group figured that it was important to diversify sources of support, believing that too close an association with any single funder might have drawbacks. While having learned well some of the rules of this particular game, however, they remained firmly focused on their primary objective – to continue their drama in order to teach other women about the dangers of AIDS and to maintain their support and caring work within the community. They wanted to move further afield and give performances on the outskirts of Mansa, but this required transport. And so they remained with the problem which had exercised them from the beginning: 'we need external assistance to do the things we want to do', whether it be in the form of transport or foodstuffs to give to those in need within the community, or the continuation of their income generating activities.[32] For all their apparent success, they remained as ever at a cross-roads, even if emboldened through their experience and the skills they had acquired.

Natweshe Development Club

The Natweshe Club was based in Lukakula, one of the cluster of villages which made up Chitamba. In the spring of 1996, a number of women living there decided to reinvigorate an earlier, abortive effort to form a women's club as a basis for income generation. As the group was in the area in which we were working, had already recruited fifteen paid up members in preparation for its relaunching, and seemed interested in community health issues as well as income generation, we asked whether they would be willing to participate in a focus group discussion about AIDS.[33] They agreed and the discussion was duly held. How much their professed interest was in hopes of using this 'angle' as a device for securing external support, or how much it was an expression of genuine concern to work around AIDS was not entirely clear.

Perceptions undoubtedly varied among participants. In the event their formal constitution included a component focusing on AIDS.

The initial focus group and the subsequent follow-up sessions generated interest among both men and women, and husbands were soon drawn into the group's activities. In respect of AIDS this reflected an admission by some women that they could not engineer the changes required on their own, Men needed to be involved, at the very least to hear the message: 'this AIDS problem can only be prevented as long as the men are brought into full co-operation'.[34] In consequence, and facilitated by members of the research team and one of the local UN volunteers, members of the group held a couples meeting to discuss AIDS.[35] Although only a small number of couples attended, it was an important innovatory development.

Husbands also got involved in the income generating activities and within a few months of the club's relaunching had come together with their wives to make bricks and construct a club house. They recognised this as an important marker of their collective resolve and collateral of sorts in respect of possible external support. The promise of assistance was forthcoming near the end of 1996 when the local UNDP team decided to adopt them, intrigued by their couples meeting and seeing them as a potential model of an energetic, community-based anti-AIDS cum income generating initiative. The local branch of the Zambia Planned Parenthood Association also cast an interested eye upon them as a group capable of revitalising its efforts to encourage the use of contraceptives in Chitamba.[36]

As these developments unfolded, the group itself evolved, as reflected in its change of name, from the Natweshe Social Club to the Natweshe Development Club. A visit to the club by the Permanent Secretary of the Province and the town mayor was reported in the national press.[37] A representative of the Zambia Popular Theatre Alliance gave them an afternoon of training and encouraged them to use drama as a tool for AIDS education.[38] But then things began to go wrong. Promised a grant of seeds and fertiliser, the Club had started to prepare their common field. However, the supplies did not materialise – not an unknown problem in the agricultural experience of the province, but devastating none the less. The top dressing came too late to save the crop and the yield was extremely disappointing.[39] Even so they persevered.

The women then began to grow restless. Elections at the time of the name change had brought men onto the executive and the agenda seemed to slip away from the women, with emphasis on an activity (farming) about which they now had second thoughts. One of the leading lights of the group from its origins was a woman who, while always entertaining the possibility of the women maintaining a collective garden, preferred them to embark on tailoring, an activity in which she already had some experience. A number of the other women shared this interest. There began to be an undercurrent within the group, of the women regretting having let in the men and wishing to go their own way, bolstered by frustration over what had always been a somewhat ambitious agricultural endeavour, which in the end yielded scant returns.[40]

But perhaps the decisive blow was the death of the woman whose inspiration had been central to the club's formation and who had served first as its secretary and then as its chair. Her husband had died earlier at the very time the club was finding its feet. It is possible that these were AIDS deaths, and even if this remained only a matter of conjecture, it made all the more poignant the fortunes of the group in respect of its objectives. Given the club's difficulties, the loss of the spark and direction that she had provided were deeply felt. 'When she died', said one of the women,'the club died with her'.[41]

Local UNDP workers tried to encourage the group further. Two of its members were invited to attend the same training session in peer education toward the end of 1997 as that attended by the Muchinka women. However, skills acquired were not put into practice, and UN volunteers began to form the view that the group was not serious and merely wanted hand-outs.[42] For their part, members of the group grumbled (perhaps with some justification) that their distance from the district and provincial offices discouraged close contact and that they were neglected compared with other groups (such as the Muchinka women).[43]

Lisach Women's Club

The third group, the Lisach Women's Club, is a very different case from the other two.[44] Situated in a village on the outskirts of town, close to the Mansa River and a little to the east of Chitamba, it was the inspiration of a couple living at the original mission station of the CMML (Christian Missions in Many Lands) church in Mansa. Formed in 1997, Lisach was named in memory of the man's mother, who had expressed her Christian conviction through the work she had done over many years for the local community. In significant degree, the club was an extension of her work and expressed similar conviction, although it had no official association with the church. Her son took on the project after being made redundant from his job in a parastatal, not as a source of personal income but as a genuine expression of his religious faith.

Lisach was very much a creature of the AIDS epidemic, having grown out of the couple's concern over the way that AIDS was wreaking havoc on families in the area, leaving an increasing number of widows and orphans, who often found it difficult to cope: 'our target group is widows, those most vulnerable to marriage problems, divorce and early child bearing without husbands. These have many problems. The aim is to empower such women'. However, membership was also open to others, and in 1998, eight married women were included among its thirty members.[45] Women were recruited to the club to learn new skills and to be recipients of information, including that related to HIV. Much of the instruction was carried out by the couple themselves. Income generation was a major activity, with members routinely engaged in sewing, knitting and the making of crafts and foodstuffs.

The club had benefited from a donation of sewing machines and other supplies from missionaries via the CMML church and had also received advice from American Peace Corps volunteers about how to obtain registration and put together proposals for external assistance. One proposal had already resulted in a substantial grant from FINNIDA for the digging of a well for the surrounding community and plans were afoot for lodging another. Although some external assistance had been received, however, the club was not dependent upon it. However, any conclusion that it was self-sustaining would gloss over the very substantial contribution of the couple, and particularly the husband, who carried out training and marketing and wrote the proposals for funding.

Evaluation of group experiences

What makes a group 'work'? Strengths at the level of organisation

On the basis of only a few cases, conclusions about criteria for success of community-based AIDS initiatives must remain tentative. Still they provide some useful insight.

In terms of longevity and the meeting of formal objectives, issues of leadership, members' commitment and (financial) viability may be particularly important. All three groups had key individuals who brought with them vision and crucial skills. In the case of the Muchinka group, this was the woman who had belonged to an earlier drama club, who pushed so strongly for external support, demanded recognition of the real costs of their work, and so single-mindedly pursued the goals of teaching other women about AIDS and caring for those in need. However, what was particularly striking in this group was its successful transition to a new head when the first had to withdraw to care for her dying son. In contrast, the attempt to share leadership with men in the Natweshe group, while initially effective, proved difficult to sustain when the group lost the woman whose spark had illuminated its activities. As for Lisach, the man who had founded it with his wife gave hugely of his time and energy, serving as its foundation and driving force. At great personal sacrifice, he filled an essentially paternalistic role. This style of leadership proved highly effective in the initial stages but in the long run could limit the scope of empowerment formally aspired to.

A sense of commitment and of mutual support was regarded by members of the Muchinka drama group as crucial to its longevity. As one of its leaders said with elegant simplicity, 'the group works because we are able to work together. Even if a problem arises we are able to discuss it and solve it ourselves. It is important to be united in all the things we do'.[46] But they also employed mechanisms to facilitate commitment, such as following up a member's absence and fining her if she missed two meetings or, when they received their first grant, dividing themselves into smaller groups to manage its use in order to ensure accountability, through co-operation and a sense of joint responsibility. They brought new members into the group on probation and had 'disqualified' several because of their 'negative feelings' towards those with AIDS.[47] They insisted that members accept that the core purpose of the group was to do work around AIDS and not to benefit from income generation: 'income generation is there to support, but drama is most important'.[48] They also helped one another: 'if a member is ill or has a sick person in her household, members of the club will buy mealie meal for her'.[49]

Some of these same elements could also be found in other groups, if in different combination and perhaps to a lesser extent. Members of the Natweshe Club demonstrated their affection and respect for their chair on her death by paying a considerable proportion of the costs of transporting her body to her natal area, in the process using much of the (meagre) profit from their farming operation. As well as gaining directly from their income generating activities, members of Lisach supported two of their number who had experienced bereavements. What was particularly notable in the case of the Muchinka drama group, however, was their sense of shared responsibility. Tensions sometimes arose between members and debate over future plans could be heated; difficulties stalked their progress. However, they had been able to stick to their original purpose. As one member explained, she had joined precisely because of her admiration for the spirit of hard work and unity which the club exhibited.[50] Their example, indeed, had prompted the formation of a 'junior group' who aspired to emulate their activities.

Longevity also depended on the combination of skills, energy and time members contributed, which was in turn bound up with the relationship individuals perceived to exist between costs and benefits of group membership. In the case of the Muchinka women and the man who put his energies into the Lisach group, there was a strong spirit of voluntarism, often supported by religious faith. Indeed, while not its only basis, religious conviction remains an important motivation for community service, often displacing an individualistic and materialistic orientation. This has applied particularly in home care programmes, not just in respect of the original examples which developed in Zambia's mission hospitals, but also to many which have devolved to the community, as in Kanyama and on Zambia's Copperbelt (Blinkhoff *et al.*, 1999).

Given the costs involved and the circumstances of participants, voluntarism may have its limits, particularly for those who may hare already incurred expenses through the care or loss of a family member to AIDS. Thus, while willing to sacrifice, give of their time and dig in their pockets, the market women, in particular, were adamant about their need for further support. They recognised that *communal* gains accrued to their work and that they also gained respect and a degree of social prestige. It was energising to be applauded in the speech of the provincial permanent secretary during local World Health Day celebrations in 1998 and to have bags of maize donated to them by UNDP's resident representative. And though they grumbled, they also recognised that they had indeed received considerable support in training and advice from the district Medical Office and UN volunteers. In many respects this was a well-endowed and well-serviced group. However, they articulated a need for deeper support which could ultimately be self sustaining and, by giving them greater income security, make it possible for them to *afford* to give more freely of their time, as well as directly support their AIDS work. This was an ambitious objective, and though far from achieving it, they had a clear understanding of what was required.

In the other two groups, the balance was different. They were primarily income generating groups, which incorporated some AIDS education, at least for group members. They were set up with the hope of ameliorating the problem of income insecurity, in one case specifically for those directly affected by AIDS. Their fortunes differed due to choices made and circumstances encountered, in the case of the Natweshe Club for reasons partly beyond their members' control. External assistance figured differently in the two cases. Both had aimed at self-sufficiency and had demonstrated local initiative, but greater reliance on external assistance in the case of the Natweshe Club made its shortfalls particularly stressful. As with similar ventures in other parts of the district,[51] the failure of the income generating initiative, into which much collective hope and effort had been invested, directly jeopardised the AIDS activity it was intended to support.

What benefits flow to individuals?

The legacy of the Natweshe Club seemed to have been embitterment and mistrust. More positively, the outcomes of participation in collective activity may take the form of material benefit, new skills, added knowledge or increased inner strength. In the case of AIDS, an important concern is whether spill-over effects of participation have deeper consequences, enabling members to speak more openly with their children about HIV or to negotiate changes in behaviour which entail greater personal protection.

The Muchinka women accepted that their work had both immediate and potential personal benefit. As one said, she did the work, not just for the community, but for herself, her children and her husband. Another explained that 'we help others so they will help us when needed'.[52] They were quick to acknowledge its importance in helping them to gain deeper personal knowledge about AIDS, and later, given their work for the Maximum distributors, about condoms and other contraceptives. They had learned how to take care of AIDS patients, skills which in a number of cases were put into practice in caring for their husbands or close family members. Several spoke of the importance of group support in staving off the depression, which might otherwise have attended their personal experience of AIDS.

One, who had been a beneficiary of the group's community work during the last weeks of her husband's life, had been convinced that she, too, had AIDS, since ' although the marketeers preached about using condoms, my husband had refused'. She was therefore deeply grateful for their subsequent support:

'they helped me to be less depressed by teaching me the difference between HIV and AIDS. They said that I did not have AIDS yet, although I might be carrying HIV. That was a great relief to me'. By joining the group, she felt that she was able to help others in the community, telling them the importance of positive living.[53] The husband of the group's chair in 1999 had died the previous year, whether from HIV or not she did not know, but 'from what I have learned, I am not depressed and if I am infected at least I know how to live from the knowledge I have'.[54] The decision of both women to refuse sexual cleansing had been strengthened by their involvement with the group. As one explained: 'even if my husband had not died of HIV, the person with whom I was to be cleansed might have had the virus. I would be infected'.[55]

Several of the group also said that it had helped them to talk more freely with their children. According to one, 'when a child comes and asks for a condom, I would give it to them for HIV. I trust my children, but if they are having sex, I will tell them to use a condom. It is better that they protect themselves from HIV'.[56] Not all agreed with this position, which rankled in some cases with strong Christian beliefs and a preference for abstinence before marriage. But most talked to their children about HIV, in some cases suggesting that they be tested before marriage.[57]

What about themselves and their partners? Several conceded that their very involvement in the group had been initially problematic, with husbands disapproving and having to be won over. The issue of compensation or material gain was sometimes critical in this regard: 'I managed to convince my husband because of the little things we got from poultry and a few things we were selling for the club. That did the trick'.[58] Others said that as the work of the group began to be publicly acknowledged, their husbands became more supportive and indeed more interested in the messages they were conveying.

Some had begun to talk to their husbands about these issues. As one declared, 'it is better to teach those first you are living with and then to take the message out'.[59] In spite of their familiarity with condoms through the educational work they did, however, this remained a source of unease with respect to their personal situation. One explained that the issue of condoms still brought conflict in homes, and sometimes men responded with violence when its use was demanded: 'the most difficult question we face is what ways can be taken to change their attitude over the use of condoms'.[60] However, as the record of a conversation between one of the research team and a member of the drama group illustrates, there was some change here as well:

> She initially said that she had not herself used a condom and would not think of doing so because it would mean that she was having extra-marital affairs. I then posed a hypothetical situation to her. Suppose she were to discover that her husband was having an affair with another woman. She first laughed, then looked at me and, as the conversation went on, revealed that she had in fact experienced such a situation. It had happened after she joined the drama group. She had gone out on her

business for several days, buying and selling, and on returning found a condom in the bedroom. Her first reaction was a feeling of disappointment and anger with her husband. When she confronted him, he asked for forgiveness for what had happened. After giving the matter some thought, she decided that her husband cared about her, since he had, after all, used a condom. Had she not joined the club, she said, she would have just been annoyed and disappointed about her husband's unfaithfulness. It was after this incident that she and her husband starting using condoms.[61]

Clearly there was some 'spill-over' from the prevention messages they dramatised to the way they related to partners. However, its extent was variable, as were the specifics and dynamics of their individual lives, the extent of their involvement with the group and their reflection upon its implications.

Impact of collective work on the community and general gender relations more broadly

Measurement of impact remains an area on which much outstanding work remains to be done and our study permitted only preliminary assessment in this regard. In the case of the Natweshe group and Lisach, impact was mainly internal to the group and measurable in terms of the primary goal of income generation. In contrast, the women who belonged to the Muchinka group evaluated their success not in terms of the profitability of their income generating ventures, but in respect of their ability to support those in need and the impact of their health education messages. As regards care, they were confident that they had made a contribution and frustrated that they lacked sufficient resources to do more. With respect to prevention, they believed that they could see evidence of greater AIDS awareness and some changes in behaviour in the community. They pointed to a decline in sexual cleansing and said that young girls took more care to avoid falling prey to sugar daddies; parents were refraining from marrying off their daughters for the sake of money and people were generally beginning to express more compassion for those with AIDS.[62] That this list coincided with the subjects of the plays they performed, however, suggests that their assessment may have been more aspirational than strictly accurate.

But what can be said about the nature of the activity itself and the methodology used in respect of wider changes in behaviour and indeed in the nature of gender relations? The drama which the women performed exposed the relationship between gender relations and vulnerability to infection, showing how men's behaviour puts women at risk. It went to the heart of the matter and when husbands became inquisitive about their work, as one put it,[63] it provided an opening for discussion. The fact that they were articulating a message about AIDS and gender relations, and were not merely recipients of information, as was the case with the women in Lisach, further strengthened the possibility that it would have consequences for their personal behaviour and relationships.

For all that, a question was raised from time to time about possible limitations of restricting their membership to and directing their activities at women. Early in the group's existence, members justified this approach through the argument that women's misinformation or lack of information needed to be addressed so that they could more adequately protect their children: 'women are the ones who like their children to get married before they go for a test and who like cleansing' (or at least permit these things to occur and yet could be a force for change). However, it was also, they said, because 'women are victims of AIDS'.[64] Yet they acknowledged that even if they could educate women, this could only ever be a partial solution. As one put it, 'it could be that I am aware of it and the husband is reluctant to understand this. That's the only problem we are finding. The only problem lies with men'.[65] Members of their female audiences, too, felt that it was their husbands who needed to be sensitised and urged the market women to go to their places of work, in the same way that they went to places, like clinics, where women were gathered.[66] Initially, the Muchinka women took the view that men should also be taught, but separately, perhaps by their own groups: 'men as well should be invited to their own offices for their lesson'.[67] However, subsequently men did attend their performances and in some cases told them afterwards that the message was well taken and appreciated.[68]

In the case of the Natweshe group, women's concern over their inability to bring about change on their own, and their desire for men also to hear the message, led to a different approach, with an opening up of the group to men. This facilitated the holding of the innovatory couples meeting. But AIDS became an increasingly marginal part of the group's activities and the inclusion of men had other repercussions, which seemed to dilute the solidarity of the group. While a mixed group might work in other circumstances and have important advantages, this case illustrates the difficulties which such a strategy may encounter. The market women, for their part, felt that restricting membership to women increased their unity of purpose, which was already facilitated by their relative homogeneity in terms of age, as mothers and as marketeers. This gave them a specific solidarity not just as women but as women who shared particular social characteristics. On this basis they could speak more freely about the gender issues they faced than perhaps was the case with members of Lisach, who, though gaining important economic skills and income, were more passive recipients of a programme established on their behalf, than agents pushing against the boundaries of the beliefs and behaviours which confined them.

The Muchinka market women relished their relative independence. They received advice and external support – and indeed demanded it – but wished to be beholden to none but themselves. It was this methodology of group formation and operation which emboldened, indeed empowered, them, and caused others to respect them. In the case of their drama, the very nature of their AIDS work served to highlight the link between gender relations and AIDS, both within the community and within their own lives. They had gone through a collective learning process, enhanced by the episodes of training they had received, but also generated by their own deliberations and reflections, which provided them with tools and the increased confidence to speak out to others and implement changes in their lives. This did not imply a transformation of gender relations either in their own lives or in the wider community. Nor did it even ensure protection in all cases. But it was consistent with such deeper changes.

This effect was perhaps less pronounced in respect of the community care and support work which they carried out, which reinforced rather than challenged the existing gender division of labour, conforming as it did to the expectation that it is women who take responsibility for care. Yet the fact that they initiated and conducted it on their own terms strengthened them as a group and as individuals. In this sense, it promoted an image of women as strong and highly capable in their own right.

Conclusions

The positive qualities of the women's drama group should not serve to overstate the inherit weaknesses it also exhibited and the difficulties its members faced. For the group's experience also highlights the problems of community action in settings where AIDS itself debilitates physically and psychologically and causes severe economic hardship. Such communities are resource rich in the personal and collective skills and strengths of their members. But groups which emerge with a conviction that they must do something for themselves, their neighbours and their families cannot do it all. The task is far too great. The call for support which was made throughout by the women's drama group was not for handouts, nor was it evidence of donor dependence. It was a genuine expression of existing need, both for income security and for AIDS interventions. The successes and failures of all three groups demonstrate the difficulties as well as the possibilities of moving forward. But as the case of the marketeers demonstrates, it is a rocky path, on which groups seem so often to be at a cross-roads, so that in spite of motivation and past success, they can easily fall with the next step, or limp forward only with difficulty, because the resource foundation on which they rest is so fragile.

Notes

1   An earlier account of AIDS activities in Mansa, which deals with two of the groups discussed in this chapter, the Muchinka Women's Drama Club and the Natweshe club, can be found in Bujra and Baylies (1999).

2   Women, of course, are not a homogeneous group and the importance of divisions among them must also be heeded.

3   The research at this site was carried out by a team of individuals, all of whom made

significant contributions. Lillian Mushota, with the assistance of Felix Posta, carried out an initial visit to Mansa in June 1995. In October 1995, they returned, accompanied by Carolyn Baylies. In November 1995, the research was progressed by Carolyn Baylies and Tashisho Chabala. Arnold Kunda and Anastasia Mwewa carried out the base-line survey and assisted Carolyn Baylies and Tashisho Chabala with the first set of focus group discussions and Tashisho Chabala with the second set. Arnold Kunda continued to monitor the situation through the end of January 1997. Tashisho Chabala made follow-up visits in December 1997 and July 1998. Carolyn Baylies and Tashisho Chabala conducted a final follow-up in September 1999. Special thanks should be given to officers at district and provincial levels working in the AIDS fields and, in particular, to Elias Maarugu, who gave crucial assistance to the project in its first 2 years.

4 The figure for those aged 15–19 was estimated to be 16 per cent, for those 20–29, 29 per cent, and for those 30–44, 14 per cent (NASTLP, n.d.).

5 Figures are based on our base-line survey in Chitamba.

6 Mansa focus group, Muchinka market women, 14 April 1996, facilitator, T. Chabala.

7 Research diary, T. Chabala, 26 November 1995. The practice has been made illegal for those in civil marriages and is soundly condemned by many in the country. The other members of this group were aware of their legal rights but had feared being 'bewitched' had they asserted their claims.

8 Sexual cleansing has been officially discouraged for some years in favour of non-sexual alternatives; in some cases where it still occurs, traditional courts have required participants to first have an HIV test.

9 Of those included in our base-line survey, about one-third gave their ethnicity as Bemba, 30 per cent as Aushi, the local ethnic group, and a further 20 per cent as an ethnic group from elsewhere in Luapula.

10 In the Chitamba sample, 29 per cent listed their main source of income as farming, 28 per cent as wage work and 23 per cent as self employed trade.

11 Even so the situation in Mansa district is much less dire than elsewhere in Luapula. Across the province as a whole 72 per cent were categorised as 'core poor' in the mid 1990s on the basis of the government's own indicators (Seketeni *et al.*, 1995).

12 Group discussion, civil servants, Mansa, 12 April, 1996.

13 In 1995, a strong programme was in place centred around Mbereshi Hospital and funded by a Danish church-based NGO, involving the co-ordination of nine local anti-AIDS clubs, counselling services, a home-based care programme with fifty clients, training of community volunteers, support for drama groups and health education. At Mambilima's health facility, connected with the CMML church, home-based support and an orphans' programme were in place as well as a monthly discussion group for those who were living with HIV (Research diary, C. Baylies, 25 October 1995; 30 October 1995).

14 Interview, District AIDS Officer, October 1995. At the end of the decade, however, a branch of Youth Alive was set up in Mansa, centred around the Catholic Cathedral (but non-denominational in intent and membership), which showed promise of capturing the enthusiasm of the youth (Research diary, C. Baylies, 8 September 1999).

15 Mansa has been one of several sites in Zambia to which UNDP has sent a series of international volunteers, generally from other African countries. In Mansa these have typically been slotted in as provincial level IEC specialists, but have characteristically focused their endeavours on AIDS activities in Mansa District, and more specifically Mansa town. Their work has been supplemented by Zambians appointed as local or national UN volunteers. UNDP has not always funded specific projects but the programme has served as a strong basis for generating donor support, for example from Germany and Norway.

16   Muchinka Teen Centre, progress reports, July–September 1993; January–December 1994.
17   Research diary, T. Chabala, 25 May 1996.
18   Research diary, C. Baylies, 26 October 1995.
19   Research diary, T. Chabala. 30 May 1996.
20   Text of speech of Mr Mubanga, Permanent Secretary, Luapula Province, 2 December 1996, Mansa Central Market.
21   Research diary, T. Chabala, 29 April 1996.
22   Research diary, T. Chabala, 29 April 1996; group discussion, Mansa, 10 May 1996, facilitator, T. Chabala.
23   Research diary, A. Kunda, 9 July 1997.
24   Research diary, T.Chabala, 8 August 1996.
25   Research diary, A. Kunda, 23 August 1996; C. Baylies, 29 August 1996.
26   Group discussion, C. Baylies Research diary, 31 August 1996.
27   Group discussion, C. Baylies Research diary, 31 August 1996.
28   Research diary, A. Kunda, 11 December 1996; 19 January 1997; at the same time they received a much smaller amount from the research project, in recognition of the value of the work they were doing. This they put into the bank.
29   Letter, A. Kunda, 20 July 1998; Research diary, T. Chabala, 16 July 1998.
30   Letter, A. Kunda, 20 July 1998.
31   Research diary, T. Chabala, 16 August 1998.
32   Meeting of Muchinka Women's Drama Group, 9 September 1999.
33   Research diary, C. Baylies, 15 April 1996.
34   Group discussion, Lukakula, 30 August 1996, facilitator, T. Chibala.
35   Research diary, T. Chabala, 8 August 1996.
36   Correspondence, A. Kunda, 25 October 1996; December 1996.
37   Correspondence, A. Kunda, December 1996.
38   Research diary, A. Kunda, 16 January 1997.
39   Research diary, A. Kunda, 13 January 1997; 19 January 1997; 21 January 1997 and correspondence 25 January 1997.
40   Correspondence, A. Kunda, 20 July 1998; T. Chabala report, 'Analysis of Women's Clubs in Mansa,' July 1998; Research diary, T. Chabala 21 July 1998.
41   Correspondence, A. Kunda, 20 July 1998; T. Chabala report, 'Analysis of Women's Clubs in Mansa,' July 1998; Research diary, T. Chabala, 18 July 1998.
42   Research diary T. Chabala, 16 July 1998; 22 July 1998.
43   Research diary, T. Chabala, 18 July 1998; 21 July 1998.
44   Research diary, T. Chabala, 19 July 1998; Interviews, 8 September 1999 and 9 September 1999, Mansa.
45   Research diary, T. Chabala, 19 July 1998.
46   Interview 5, 8 September 1999.
47   Interview 1, 8 September 1999.
48   Interview, 4, 8 September 1999.
49   Interview, 1, 8 September 1999.
50   Research diary, T. Chabala, 20 July 1998.
51   Research diary, C. Baylies, 8 September 1999.
52   Interviews, 1 and 2, 8 September 1999.
53   Research diary, T. Chabala, 20 July 1998.
54   Interview, 5, 8 September 1999.
55   Interview, 5, 8 September 1999.
56   Interview, 1, 8 September 1999.
57   Research diary, T. Chabala, 20 July 1998.
58   Research diary, T. Chabala, 17 July 1998.
59   Interview, 5, 8 September 1999.
60   Correspondence, A. Kunda, 12 November 1996.

61 Research diary, T. Chabala, 14 July 1998.
62 Research diary, T. Chabala, 20 July 1998.
63 Research diary, T. Chabala, 17 July 1998.
64 Focus group, Women's drama group, 5 June 1996, facilitator, T. Chabala.
65 Research diary, C. Baylies, 31 August 1996.
66 Research diary, T. Chabala, 8 August 1996.
67 Research diary, C. Baylies, 31 August 1996.
68 Correspondence, A. Kunda, 11 December 1996.

8 AIDS activism in Dar es Salaam: many struggles; a single goal

Janet Bujra and Scholastica N. Mokake

All over Africa, the terrible calamity of AIDS has forced people out of isolation induced by fear, stigma and blame, and into collective action. Out of despair comes the resolution that 'something must be done' to confront an impending epidemic threatening life and livelihoods alike. AIDS associations have multiplied, often in consequence of indigenous initiatives. It is one such association, WAMATA[1] in Tanzania, on which we focus here, tracking its progress from local self-help support group to highly professional national organisation with major branches in six urban areas, a network of over fifty smaller branches throughout the country, and a youth wing (WAMATA *Newsletter*, January–March 1999).[2] Initially, a response to early deaths amongst the better-off and more educated in Dar es Salaam, its work is now focussed mainly on the impoverished (and amongst these, particularly women and youth). Its major activities are home-based care and counselling, support groups for the affected, preventative education and advocacy. Three issues are highlighted in analysis of this pioneering development: the broader debate about the role of national-level NGOs[3] in contemporary development practice and AIDS work; the way class and gender configure in NGO activity; and the dilemmas posed by the professionalising process in AIDS activities. Our aim here is social analysis, not organisational evaluation.

The NGO debate

The burgeoning of indigenous and externally-led AIDS NGOs in Africa has taken place in the context of state withdrawal from the very services (health and education) crucial to coping with and stemming the epidemic. This 'rolling back of the state' is in its turn the consequence of economic and political 'liberalisation', encompassed in structural adjustment packages forced on African governments in order to secure debt relief. As international financial institutions (IFIs) were imposing these terms, they were also celebrating alternatives to the state in what was seen as its antithesis, civil society. Indigenous NGOs were seen as a key element in this new development paradigm, more cost-effective, more participatory, more efficient and more inclusive than top-heavy organs of the state. (The implications of this debate for Tanzania are reviewed in Mercer, 1999). If neoliberalism embraced the NGO sector, so too did many radicals, for whom it appeared to promise an emancipatory agenda for the oppressed (Edwards and Hulme, 1995; Pearce, 2000). AIDS activism thus flourished in a broad welcoming climate of international regard and prospects for funding.

The optimistic view has recently come into question. IFIs now concede that state regulation may be crucial to framing development (World Bank, 1997, 2000). Critical questions are also posed by more radical thinkers for whom the emancipatory promise of the non-state sector is now in doubt. Some see NGOs as institutions exploited by state and IFIs alike to fill in the welfare gaps left by state withdrawal (Robinson, 1998; Commins, 1999; Mercer, 1999). The acclaimed cost-effectiveness of NGO provision may be explained as the appropriation of voluntary labour (Thomas, 1998). Some argue that states fear the very empowerment of civil society that indigenous NGOs are claimed to deliver and are quick to muzzle and constrain them (Mercer, 1999, referring to the Tanzanian case).

Critical research into the promised emancipatory agenda of the NGO has sometimes revealed ambiguous outcomes. On the one hand the burgeoning of non-state associations may create openings and support for those previously excluded or marginalised: women, ethnic or religious minorities, the homeless or street children. More cynically it is argued that NGOs provide opportunities for new kinds of 'elite formation', rather than empowering 'the poor' (Kiondo, 1993; Dozon and Chabal, 1999; Mercer, 1999; Trivedy, 1999). In relation to AIDS activism, Setel has quoted a common view in Tanzania, that 'AIDS is business' (Setel, 1996: 1176).

Class and gender dynamics

Here we argue for a more ambiguous picture. To assert that processes of class formation[4] find expression in the creation and activities of NGOs is not to imply, in psychologistic or moralistic terms, that NGO activists have 'ulterior motives', are 'greedy' or 'on the make', even though that is how their actions may look to others less fortunately placed. Many of those involved are driven by deep concern for others and the courage to defy convention in pursuing their commitment. Moreover, their collective work has often been groundbreaking in bringing help to the destitute, the dying and the oppressed. It is *analytically* useful to define NGO workers in class terms, as members of a petty-bourgeoisie aiming to express and consolidate its position relative to other class fractions. This may take symbolic as well as practical forms.

There are parallels between the burgeoning of welfare NGOs in developing countries and the philanthropic movements seen in Europe and America in the late nineteenth century. Philanthropy, in its zeal to uplift, rescue, enlighten and modernise the working class, entered into dangerous class alliances at the same time that it symbolically marked its distance from the 'lower orders'. Philanthropy was often motivated by fear – of political unrest or of contagion (in the modern era AIDS provides a parallel – it is no respecter of class boundaries). Nineteenth century philanthropy took hold in a context of capitalist consolidation, but similar developments may be cited from present-day developing countries where class divisions cut deep (e.g. India: Caplan, 1978). The contemporary African case looks at first sight very different, for here class boundaries are ill-defined and shifting, and there is little surplus wealth to be diverted into charity as a mode of class control. Here, the emergence of welfare NGOs represents the privatisation of the provision of public goods. Those who run NGOs would formally have been employed by the state (funded through taxes and foreign aid); now they must freelance to earn their keep. The object of their class concern (the poor, the powerless, the sick and uneducated) cannot pay for services previously provided in a limited way through the public purse, or for their innovative expansion. This petty bourgeoisie must thus transform itself. They become private entrepreneurs touting for funds in the world aid market.

It is no accident that these developments (philanthropy, charity, NGO activity) are often gendered: they express the marginalisation of women at higher class levels. In the phase of international hyper-enthusiasm for NGOs, the virtuous claim was that such organisations would address gender inequity or at least be more gender sensitive than agents of the state. The rhetoric has been powerful, but reality is more variable (Goetz, 1997; Harrison, 1997; Jackson, 1997; Trivedy, 1999). 'Gender awareness' rarely includes confronting men's behaviour; conversely women with differing class interests may not exhibit solidarity even when engaged in collective action. Does this apply in AIDS work too?

The professionalisation of AIDS work

There is also debate about the impact of routinisation, institutionalisation and bureaucratisation on the capacity of NGOs to deliver. Here, some of the discursive and practical struggles of addressing the AIDS problem in Europe and America resonate with African dilemmas, though the context is very different. Where AIDS predominantly affected gay men, models of peer-working were often developed, based on the success of gay men's own organisations. Deverell (1997) notes the ambiguous role of the professional outreach worker in such contexts. The credibility of peer workers in the field was established through being part of 'the scene' – a risk-taking equal. However, workers also needed legitimacy as professionals, and this entailed a distancing from 'clients', claims to status, adherence to a code of professional ethics and to possession of 'expert, systematised, and theoretical... knowledge' (op. cit.: 152). However, workers needed to be both peer and professional in order to survive, and the two roles often clashed with one another. Gay men had often regarded professionals with suspicion in the past, whilst the transgressive association of this work with sexuality put the workers' 'professionalism' in question.

In Africa, the context is very different, given that all sexually-active adults are potentially at risk. However, professionalisation is again at issue, this time more clearly exposing class relations. Activism in Africa often begins as self-help, like gay activism in the West. In confronting the unprecedented and ever-expanding crisis of AIDS, the voluntary self-help group is quickly overwhelmed. In seeking funding, devising ways to approach benefactors and recruiting paid workers it is forced to routinise its operations. For some, this expansion becomes an additional or even alternative motive for action, an opportunity for income, for a career, for class mobility. The question is whether the professionalisation it embodies also creates a disabling distance between those who suffer and those who ease suffering: the former becoming 'clients' and dependants rather than fellow human beings at risk. Women are disproportionately drawn into this work as stereotypical carers of the sick, but now they too are drawn into the professionalisation process. Becoming involved in helping those who are moral outcastes might be contagious, putting their professionalisation in question. The transgressive nature of the work may jar with what women are supposed to know and how they are supposed to behave.

Evaluation of the activities of AIDS organisations needs to be set in this critical moment of change – in an international climate where civil society is promoted against the state, and locally, in ongoing struggles around class and gender. All of these contested developments are manifest in AIDS activism in Dar es Salaam.

Dar es Salaam and the epidemic

The AIDS epidemic did not begin in the capital city. Almost certainly it was brought there by migrants and travellers from the first area to be affected – Kagera in the far north-west. The first cases were noted in Dar by the mid-1980s. A decade later the levels of prevalence of HIV were higher in Dar es Salaam Region than anywhere else (NACP, 1998b: 19). Between 1995 and 1997 prevalence rose from 13.5 to 14.8 per cent (NACP, 1999: 16, 19)[5]. AIDS has now become the commonest cause of death in the capital (NACP, 1999: 6).

Like other heavily affected regions in Tanzania, Dar es Salaam has a large number of AIDS NGOs – twenty-five were counted in 1997, amongst which the two best-known were WAMATA and the Society for Women and AIDS in Tanzania (SWAAT). Several other organisations had extended pre-existing work with youth, medical research or religious proselytisation to the AIDS field (Msaky and Kisesa, 1997).

With a population of over two million, the city is growing fast[6]. Rapid urban growth has meant an influx of rural people who rarely settle permanently in the capital. Women as well as men form part of the migratory flow. Both men and women struggle to survive; the majority subsist ingeniously, though at a low level, through small-scale trade and petty production of goods and services. They live in crowded houses in dusty streets, in neighbourhoods full of the noise of life and commercial activity.

We have here social settings characterised by high geographic mobility, with a population weighted towards the most sexually active age group, where individuals are making new lives away from the constraints and support of kin and elders, and where social conventions to contain relations between the sexes and generations and to mediate the babel of contrasting customs and patterns of behaviour are rooted in shallow soil. At the extreme, life in the poorer neighbourhoods of Dar es Salaam goes on in highly sexualised contexts where risk and survival hunt together. An extract from first hand observation in 1997[7]:

> During the night, people at Hyena Ground (in Manzese) become so many... People drink to the extent of doing and shouting a lot of things without being aware of what they are doing. Sexuality and sex are displayed openly, especially by the prostitutes who are there renting rooms and waiting for customers. There are times when the slum houses, special for short time renting, are too few for the number of customers and each customer has to book his time from the house owners... After returning from school, children from poorer families come here to sell cooked food brought from their homes to earn money for their families. Mostly young girls between the ages of 10 and 12, they arrive at around 6 p.m. and work to 10 p.m.... we saw many young and old men trying to seduce them by offering money which would cover the total sales of food... and give them the chance to have sex with the girls. One man was overheard to say, 'I'm giving you this money to give mama so that we can make love before you have to get off home'.
>
> (J. Lutimba and J. Mwabuki, 1997)

In other areas where we carried out observations, sexual commerce was less openly on display, but other factors lent risk to everyday life: men's greater purchasing power than women; women's greater need ('women are selling the disease and men with their money buy it', was one man's comment)[8]; men's violence and sexual brutality and women's fear and sense of powerlessness in situations where social support is limited; young men's inability to marry given dire economic circumstances; and the sexual abuse of young girls by older men (often also a form of class exploitation). There are constraints over such behaviour; people do not live in a state of normlessness. Even in the poorest areas there are institutions which express collective values of 'proper' behaviour: churches, mosques, local leaders, ethnic associations, parents struggling to keep families together and protect their children – but their reach is less secure than in settled rural areas. Neither does impoverishment mean ignorance. Every adult in Dar es Salaam knows that AIDS kills and that it is transmitted largely through sexual relations.

Despite the seemingly obvious association between AIDS and poverty in

Dar es Salaam, AIDS activism was not generated in such contexts. It came rather out of the leafy suburbs and the campus, the social milieu of the educated and comfortably-off, those whose world was shattered by the realisation that their income, their modern knowledge and familiarity with scientific facts could not protect them from this invisible killer. Accounts from two activists, both children of University teachers, illustrate the compelling impact of personal affliction on the decision to become involved. In both cases a sibling died of AIDS – these were amongst the first recorded cases in the capital. The bereaved were still struggling to make sense of how the victim had become infected. In one case they blamed socially unacceptable sexual liaisons – adultery, but in a context of oppressive family relations that had led to a forced marriage. In both cases their misfortune brought them cruelly into the public eye. As one said, '(my brother) was a known person, he was an artist, he used to draw in the newspapers, everybody knew he was sick'. People had just begun to hear about AIDS and they were overcome with a morbid curiosity, which quickly turned into stigmatisation of the sick and their relatives. 'In Africa…when you hear somebody is sick you must go and see the person. So they will come at home to visit us and you welcome them with 'soda' (soft drinks) and maybe they are afraid to use your glasses – and then you feel bad'. The speaker was still at school and she found school friends avoiding her: 'they don't want to study with me because I have a brother who has HIV'.

It was bereaved men and women like this, together with the sick and their friends and relatives, who formed the initial nucleus of an association dedicated to fighting AIDS. It was a far-seeing and educated woman who put the knowledge of suffering in her homeland together with observation of support groups in North America to envision the idea of WAMATA. Theresa Kaijage was a lecturer at the Institute of Social Welfare who had lost relatives and friends.[9] She approached others who were affected and asked for their help in setting up a support group. Established in 1989, it ran at first on voluntary help and with injections of cash and kind from its founder and supporters. 'A certain Roman Catholic Brother…gave us his room to use free (as an office)'.[10] When meetings were held, one or another 'will bring a crate of soda'. And the founder 'used her own car' to transport a sick man home.

If this association sprang from the better-off and supported them in seeking treatment and comfort for their relatives, it also immediately reached out to the poor and the destitute – widows whose husbands had died of AIDS and had no money to feed their children, sick women who could not afford accommodation. Kaijage approached one of the public hospitals for permission to visit those diagnosed with AIDS. If such people were then transmuted into 'clients', the process was one which challenged convention on both sides and in which the rules were made up as they went along.

Three young volunteers undertook to visit a man who was dying in hospital and whose family had abandoned him. He discovered that his relatives had announced he was already dead (and buried by the City Council) and that they had mourned 3 days for him as was customary. The dying man begged the volunteers to take him home to prove that he was still alive. Mama Theresa agreed, in the belief that this would set his mind at rest. Returning home, he had the psychological satisfaction of shaming his relatives by accusing them of abandoning him and lying about his death. He then returned to hospital with his 'new friends', dying a few days later. WAMATA were forced to bury him. In this creative handling of the case, WAMATA broke the silence of denial about AIDS, demonstrated its commitment to the dying and showed how they could be treated with compassion and respect.

From self help to professionalisation

The initial impetus to voluntary collective action could not survive the encounter with the magnitude of the AIDS problem. As early as 1991, the Dar group was caring for:

> 'forty-nine people with AIDS; milk is provided for seventy-two children; forty-seven widows are being supported; eleven people with HIV infection have been taken home; and school fees for fifty-four primary school and twenty secondary school pupils are being provided...funeral arrangements had been made for twenty-five people... and financial support was being given to eleven people'
>
> (Kaijage, 1991: 12).

A decade later it is possible to evaluate the extent to which the practice of WAMATA has been marked by pressures to routinise the charismatic impulse which first sparked it into existence. The most potent of these pressures has flowed from the need to generate funds.

Once volunteers build up some expertise and knowledge, their skills become too valuable to lose, and given the scale of the AIDS crisis, there is a pressing need to extend the skills base through processes of formal training. This immediately requires a more formal designation of roles and task descriptions and payment for work. The long term commitment to pay salaries is beyond the resources of voluntary effort and bids to secure funding become necessary. This process imposes its own constraints, as funders must be wooed with promises to fulfil objectives which are not always the same as those of the bidders. In Tanzania the need for funding coincides with the contraction of the state, and whilst organisations like WAMATA were clearly taking on a public welfare role, state resources were unavailable. Some funds could be generated within the organisation (see below), but they were woefully inadequate compared with need. Only foreign donors had the kind of money required. To approach foreign donors required official permission, and WAMATA had to be formally registered to proceed. This was achieved in 1990, and WAMATA was thereafter licensed to operate under the surveillance of the National AIDS Control Programme. Through the process of getting official approval, WAMATA were in effect designated a task which would relieve the public purse: 'we were told, maybe you concentrate on the home base (home-based care), because the hospitals they are full of people – it's better these people should be taken care of at home'.

WAMATA was successful in its bids to foreign donors. Over the years it has been supported by the Danish aid organisation, DANIDA, NORAD and several other international agencies.[11] Whilst there is still a significant element of voluntary labour put into WAMATA (some 'clients' become volunteer peer counsellors, and the branch chairs and their executive committees are volunteers) the major expenses of running the association depend on awards from external funders.

The promise of funding allowed WAMATA to shift from reliance on unpaid volunteers and to create the role of professional paid AIDS 'counsellor'. For the original volunteers 'it was just using our common sense', but now 'we came to learn that there are some ethics'. There were also techniques, which could facilitate interaction, and ways to support people to discover their HIV status; there were ways of telling people bad news and helping them to live positively thereafter. How the new WAMATA counsellors learned all this illustrates the productive networking that goes on in Africa. Mama Theresa assiduously invited influential contacts to their meetings and then enlisted their help. They were first offered training by the USAID-funded AIDSCOM project in Dar es Salaam. Then some of them were funded by DANIDA to go to Zambia to learn from the home-based programme run by Chikankata hospital. They visited sick people with the teams of doctors in that scheme, listening to how it was done. Then they went to talk with TASO, the organisation set up by Noerine Kaleeba in Uganda (Kaleeba, 1991). 'We learnt a lot from them'. WAMATA practice evolved, focussing attention not only on the sick, but 'you deal with the whole family... you need to know about the other family members, if there is a grandmother who is taking care, if there are children – are they going to school?' (see also Kaijage, 1991: 12).

In the new professional ethics, the issue of confidentiality was paramount but problematic. It clashed with local cultural norms – 'we normally share' – and with the need to protect those needing information in order to protect themselves. Usually this meant the sexual partners of those who tested positive – and here the practice became one of persuasion – impressing on the client the gravity of continued unprotected intercourse and supporting them to disclose the truth to relevant others. Another example underlines WAMATA's commitment to whole families (an account based on interview with a WAMATA counsellor):[12]

A woman client had a daughter who was also HIV positive. The daughter had a tiny baby, very sick and small. When the client died, the family sent for *shangazi*[13] – her husband's sister, an elderly woman from rural Songea. *Shangazi* saw that there was little hope for her dying niece, but she expected to rescue the baby. When counsellors went on a home visit they found *shangazi* sucking bloody mucous out of the child's mouth and nose to help it breathe. They were horrified (given the danger of infection) and told her gently that she shouldn't do this – they would bring some drops and other medicine for the child. On speaking to the child's mother they discovered that *shangazi* had not been told about the HIV status of her niece and that the baby was probably infected too, though all the other family members knew. The counsellors asked: 'How can she be a carer when she doesn't know?' The girl agreed reluctantly that they must tell *shangazi*.

(J. Bujra, Fieldnotes, 1995)

Confidentiality might also conflict with the drive to have WAMATA known and to break the silence around AIDS. 'In 1991 we had our pick-up and it was written 'WAMATA'. So when you go for home visits people are asking 'What is WAMATA?'. However, soon, clients told us, 'please don't come with the car to the house'. So we used to park far away and walk to the house'. If people knew that the sick had AIDS they would be stigmatised, suffer avoidance from fellow tenants and maybe even lose their accommodation.

Becoming a counsellor meant learning to be a professional and doing the job according to agreed rules of procedure. It was a job which brought men and women into direct and daily contact with the sick and the desperate and for some this was its major reward, giving them the opportunity to be useful. However, the pay was limited. A limited career ladder began to be erected within the organisation as it expanded, with some staff specialising in training and recruiting, or more administrative roles. Inevitably this took them away from interacting with clients: 'now I'm doing a lot of office work and report writing, job descriptions for counsellors… a lot of training'. They felt the loss and were gratified when clients continued to approach them for their advice. As workers progressed and consolidated their position they became aware that there was a hierarchy of professionals – there were those who were hired in on a part-time basis as medical staff and whose pay was much higher, compared with 'us who are there everyday, doing a lot! then get paid little'.

As workers were 'professionalised', so too was the organisation. Here the donors had a shaping influence:

When we wrote a proposal to DANIDA…they looked at it and they say, 'This is too much! You want to do everything and you cannot!' They say sit down and think what you want to do. So we say we can not – without the skills of how to put it, how to even write the proposal. So we had to hire a consultant.

At the beginning we did not even know. Somebody said, 'What is your mission statement?' – all these things are new, we don't know. When we started we did not have the mission statement.

Designing plans to the satisfaction of donors meant specifying objectives and time periods in advance, not dealing creatively with situations as they arose. Some donors were prepared to give money without controlling its expenditure, but understandably most were insistent on tight budgets and accounting. WAMATA and other AIDS organisations report that donor generosity has diminished over the last few years. An official of SWAAT commented that donors no longer fund free medicines even though a local consultant provides his services free: 'And those who come to us are the very poorest people!' Nor would donors now fund organisational initiatives such as calling all the SWAAT branches for an annual meeting. Funding for the material support which WAMATA used to provide to clients is also less available and donors have adopted the view that handouts create dependency. One donor was happier to fund a scheme in which women's groups were offered revolving loans – a scheme which Kaijage says was unsuccessful: 'Some donor agencies feel disappointed by this failure to 'revolve' the funds, but it is unrealistic. It is not because the participants have not tried. It is very hard to generate a surplus, enough to pay the original money' (1993: 273).

In this climate, a reversion to self-help is forced upon organisations – though this may also constitute a 'performance' for the audience of external donors. WAMATA is a membership organisation and its members pay subscriptions to join. When sick people or their relatives approach WAMATA for help this is usually provided, but they are asked at some stage to become members:

> We wanted them to pay that membership fee so that they feel they own the organisation...that they are part of it. You know even donors, when you would ask for funds, you write proposal, they ask you what is your own contribution... [it's good] if you tell them 'our membership is 2000 people and each one pays'.

The membership fee was very low, only Sh500 (50p) but people were also asked to pay Sh500 a year subscriptions. Even then, many could not afford and had to be 'forgiven'.

Donors may also require the organisations they fund to demonstrate their efficiency through regular reporting. Organisations have had to learn what counts in such reports: a growing number of clients, outcomes which match objectives and a participatory style of working with clients that demonstrates how their views are taken into account. The production of such accounts consumes a great deal of time. WAMATA also keeps records of its patients for the government. The routinisation and bureaucratisation of AIDS work feeds on itself, paperwork creating more paperwork.

Professionalisation does not necessarily mean the stifling of initiative or working rigidly by the rule book. A 'cluster' system has developed in Dar es Salaam, in which NGOs refer clients to each other for specific needs (e.g. spiritual counselling). Rather than seeing each other as competitors, a degree of creative networking takes place between the groups. Co-operation on projects and sharing of ideas is common. SWAAT developed a project in rural Rufiji whereby older women were assisted and supported to be guardians to AIDS orphans. SWAAT approached WAMATA with the idea of trying out a similar scheme in Dar es Salaam. WAMATA was able to persuade DANIDA to fund training for some of their older women members to become 'Big Mamas'. This is now a very successful programme. When WAMATA wanted to engage their women's groups in advocacy work they approached the Tanzania Media Women's Association for assistance as they have many members trained in the law (see also Mbilinyi and Mwabuki, 1996: 3).

Clients and workers

In theory all those involved in WAMATA, the dying and those who bring succour to them, are equal as 'members' of the organisation. There is a rough justice in this view: 'any one of us may already be infected', but the reality of everyday relations is not such a level playing field, and the term 'member' often gives way to the more loaded nomenclature of 'client' (with its implication of dependency and inferiority) facing paid 'staff' with their status and privileged knowledge. Awareness of inequalities in wealth and power is a taken-for-granted feature of everyday life in Dar es Salaam, often presented in the simplistic language of 'the rich' and 'the poor' – a language used by both sides. This discourse frames the work of AIDS activists: on the one hand they are conscious of being perceived as 'rich', on the other they see themselves as amongst the 'community leaders and influential people who can influence the change process'.[14]

Members of the research team in Manzese were told by local people that: 'Most of the NGOs cater for rich people and do not care to visit low-income areas like this' – even as they observed one organisation (the Tanzania AIDS Programme) making deliveries of free or subsidised condoms, and another (the African Medical Research Foundation) reported as having come to advise people about protection.[15] When NGO activists go onto the streets, they may be identified in class terms as representatives of officialdom come to make life more difficult for those who already survive on the edges (occupying illegal kiosks, selling goods without licences, preparing food or beer in unhygienic surroundings).

Where fear is overcome, the desperate may see opportunities to grab crumbs: 'On hearing the meeting has something to do with AIDS they think that we have a lot of money and maybe they are going to get loans to start business'.[16] In their eagerness to become clients of rich patrons they are angry when clientship disappoints:

> They complain!…like when we moved into a new office… we had to put air conditioning because there is a computer. There was a donor who was ready to buy us a computer, put a telephone, put carpet…When clients came and asked for material support and we say there is none, they complained, 'So you are buying computers! Look at the carpet!''.

If the poor complain, the 'rich' are uncomfortably conscious of their views – especially those who deliberately cultivate social contiguity rather than keeping their distance.

The poor[17] may be seen as 'deserving'. One worker reported a home visit to a WAMATA client whom she was told had not eaten all day. She thought it must be because he had mouth ulcers, but he did not have them. When she questioned his wife further she found they had nothing in the house, not even maize flour for porridge. The worker was moved by pity and recommended that the family receive a small allowance to help them buy food. In another case, an AIDS patient had his legs amputated after gangrenous sores failed to heal and he could not sit up. Again the workers appreciated how his poverty exacerbated his illness and they provided him with a truss.

But the poor can also be seen as grasping and instrumental. Indeed life in the low-income areas of Dar es Salaam tends to reward such survival strategies. Workers acknowledged that clients 'sometimes pretend, when they need support. People know that if you go to M and you cry you will get [something]'. In one case a worker was called to visit the widow of a man who had died of AIDS and found only a bare bed in her house, covered with old clothing and no mattress. The widow complained of chest pains and claimed her husband's relatives had taken everything when he died. 'They know these stories', added the worker, cynically. However, at the time she was convinced and went back to the office to recommend that they purchase a mattress to help the woman. She was interrupted by the woman's neighbour, come to disclose that the woman already had a mattress, which had been hidden with the neighbour in anticipation of the visit from WAMATA. So now the organisation is less trusting, makes unannounced visits – 'we can come any day' – and seeks stratagems of its own to ward off those who exploit the system.

People in dire straits take advantage of the host of associations offering support in the capital. At SWAAT we asked how many people they were helping and were told it was three or four hundred. Could some of them also be clients of WAMATA? 'They are the same people!' At WAMATA we were told: 'You will find the same client in (SHDEPHA) (the Service, Health and Development Project for People Living with HIV/AIDS), in SWAAT…they are moving from one to another!' This instrumentalism relates not only to bids for direct support for the sick. Both SWAAT and WAMATA carry out educational work, creating and working with groups in workshops on AIDS issues. Since the people whom they want to participate are desperately poor, they offer bus fares and maybe bread and soft drinks to encourage attendance. 'You will find one day there is a meeting in WAMATA [and] there's a meeting in other places, and we give them bus fare. Maybe SWAAT are giving them more than what they are getting in WAMATA. They will go to SWAAT just to register the name and then come to WAMATA!' This is not just a matter of taking material advantage: 'it means the whole idea of group or maybe peer discussions is not in their mind… They are thinking, let me get to WAMATA before they close'.

Such meetings are important to staff and to their vision of WAMATA's 'mission' – that affected people can listen to each other, but also that they can learn from workers. 'They need more information. Once these people know how to protect themselves, they will adopt safe practices'. Whilst there is a strong commitment to 'learning from each other', workers often betray their belief that they know better. They speak of clients having 'erroneous' views and needing to receive 'corrected information'. When workers go into communities they are often addressed as *Wataalamu* or 'experts'.[18] One WAMATA counsellor described how this confused her. In a workshop the participants kept addressing her as *Ndugu Mtaalam* (comrade expert): 'I had to correct (sic) them, telling them that we were all learning from each other's experiences'.

In one area WAMATA Youth were working with groups of young men and women towards setting up an AIDS project. A plan emerged to set up an Information Centre. The WAMATA volunteers (educated young men) rationalised this in terms of their own beliefs in the efficacy of science: 'There is still a lack of accurate scientific information on care and support of people with AIDS'. They hoped that this Centre would be run by local people – 'a communal decision must come from the people themselves'. Local youth were eager, but only so long as they thought WAMATA workers would be bringing both 'information' and funding opportunities. 'Nobody was able to contribute any material towards the project…they wanted external help…The youths wanted to be trained to be peer educators, counsellors, leaders and organisers…'

The 'information' that AIDS activists impart is not only on modes of transmission and forms of protection ('I start with the basic facts of HIV'). Discussions of AIDS are highly morally charged and they are often drawn into expressing their own views. It is notable here that they put across the vision of 'modern life' to people whose mores may be very different. A WAMATA activist tells parents that they must speak openly of sexual matters to their children, despite local taboos; a youth worker tells young people that there is no shame in girls carrying condoms, and that young people need to talk to each other – 'boys and girls as friends' – when the notion of pure friendship with people of the opposite sex is an alien idea.

This can be read as a class project of uplift and enlightenment, phrased in terms of 'modern' ways of doing things.[19] Whilst it may be delivered as a message about AIDS, it can be 'heard' in quite different ways. The Information Centre was aimed at education, but the enthusiasm for its establishment related to the chance of material uplift for a few through 'training'. Similarly, within WAMATA, the transition from 'client' to 'member' offers means to enhance a person's economic position. Members can become volunteers – even very poor people who might be parents to a dying child can offer to visit other sick people in their neighbourhood. Many offer their services unstintingly and give generously of their time. They are paid a small amount to travel to the office and deliver a monthly 'report'. Whilst this is in no sense a wage for their work, it may be a significant return for the very poorest. Better-off people with full-time jobs elsewhere are also found amongst the volunteers. Such people: 'like the other incentives they are getting… because now you are a member or volunteer for WAMATA there's a seminar in Arusha and they ask, can we please go?' The expenses ('sitting allowances') paid to those who attend seminars can become a significant part of their income, especially as white collar salaries are often too low to sustain families through the month. This is the other side of the coin to the tension between volunteering and the need for recompense in a hard economic climate discussed elsewhere in this book (also Mbilinyi and Mwabuki, 1996: 3).

The AIDS organisation becomes a stage on which class relations are symbolically marked out at the same time that they are occasionally transcended. This focus on class is also an acknowledgement that differences of ethnic origin or religion are rarely at issue in the operation of AIDS organisations in Tanzania. Whilst generally conservative, even the religious organisations claim to treat all; conversely 'in WAMATA we don't have religion'.

AIDS activism as a gendered project

In an early comment on the establishment of WAMATA, Kaijage (1993: 271) remarked that: 'All the gender issues we had never tackled came up at once'. It is instructive to consider how gender issues have presented themselves within WAMATA since then. First, there is a tendency for 'gender' to mean women – and in this case women's particular vulnerability to HIV infection. Second, there are the gendered relations within the organisation itself as a set of co-operative and hierarchical arrangements. Third, there is the practice of 'clients'.

Whilst the workers in WAMATA are predominantly women – and this is an organisation with a growing but established staff – some of the key positions are held by men. All the chairs of branches are men – designated correctly as 'chairmen'. This seems to have derived from the initial need to lend credibility, in a male-dominated society, to an association moving into morally ambiguous territory. Kaijage (1993: 271) tells us that in early debates around their name she had insisted on it reflecting the love and care to be shown to the afflicted. Men objected to the 'feminine' sound of this, arguing that addressing the AIDS epidemic needed more than love – they saw it, in manly terms, as a *battle*. The name of the organisation: 'Those in the *struggle* against AIDS', thus bears the stamp of male authority.

In their review of a number of AIDS NGOs in Dar es Salaam, Mbilinyi and

Mwabuki (1996) comment that the smaller grassroots organisations are predominantly staffed by female volunteers. Larger organisations offer the opportunity for paid work and here men are more in evidence. The criteria for employment have moved beyond compassion and commitment to formal qualifications 'such as high education and work experience, where women suffer because of a legacy of gender discrimination' (Mbilinyi and Mwabuki, 1996: 3). Few men are found in caring jobs on the frontline; they tend to occupy more powerful administrative and executive positions. WAMATA was not included in Mbilinyi and Mwabuki's study; it would appear to both confirm and contradict this general view. On the one hand it is true that the Executive Director is male, as are all but two of nine National Executive Committee members. However, whilst the Director is paid, the NEC members are all volunteers. Amongst paid workers in the Dar es Salaam branch, the majority are women – ten out of fourteen. Two of the male employees are humble watchmen, one is a counsellor and the last is a doctor. As an organisation founded by a woman, and one committed to gender equality, the women staff grew with the organisation and have been nurtured and promoted within it.

Amongst the clients it would appear that women also predominate, appearing as wives of the dying (absent clients), widows, or the sick mothers of fatherless children. Women are also in the majority when WAMATA organises outreach educational campaigns or discussion workshops. The setting up of women's groups has been a particular feature of WAMATA's work, given the view that women need support to protect themselves against coercive sex and the stigma of blame they often endure (accompanied in some cases by seizure of their worldly goods by their husband's relatives after his death). There is a clear commitment within WAMATA to a gendered perspective: 'widows, the way they come and explain their problem, you switch to gender, you say this is because she is a woman, that's why she is suffering all these things'.

Female staff note that women under duress – usually compounded by lack of money and resources – find it easier to talk women counsellors: '[they think] "This is a woman, she will listen to me and she will understand what I mean"'. The assumption is of shared experiential knowledge, expressed through gender identification, but also a levelling sense of common danger, irrespective of wealth or education. Generational differences may impact on communication – one staff member commented that: 'due to my age, most elderly women took me as their child, their daughter, and built trust in me'. This is more problematic than it first appears, because generally 'daughters' do not relate authoritatively to 'mothers'. The classificatory kinship relationship is superseded by the audience defining the activist as an educated 'expert' – one, however, whom as a 'daughter' they dare to question.

Men are not absent amongst the clients of WAMATA, but they are fewer than women. Where family survival is threatened by AIDS, women (as primary carers) become the experts in survival strategies, seeking out and exploiting all channels for relief – especially those which allow them to approach other women from whom they anticipate sisterly sympathy. Workers say that men are less comfortable to own their fears and less willing to admit they have a problem (they often hide behind the guise of 'asking for a friend'). This unease may be compounded by the likelihood of facing a female counsellor. Whilst such women do not conform to men's stereotypes of 'ignorant women', their knowledge may be suspect as coming from a subordinate source (Baylies and Bujra, 1995: 195). This is a society where men inform women, not vice-versa.

Over time, WAMATA has shifted its stance from supporting women perceived as victims, to becoming advocates for women's rights. Their active women's groups are now addressed by lawyers and others on issues indirectly related to AIDS – such as women's rights in marriage and inheritance, domestic violence and sexual harassment. 'We are trying to empower these women'. In Dar es Salaam such meetings are held weekly, with audiences of over sixty coming from a variety of groups in the city, including many from the very poorest areas. They list their occupations as traders and 'housewives' with a few teachers and secretaries. The audience is appreciative and participatory, probing the speakers for further information.

Whilst promoting women's rights, WAMATA has avoided confronting men's behaviour directly, even where this puts women at risk. It is not that men's greater social power is not recognised. One staff member recalled an atypical case where the woman of the house was the main breadwinner. Following suspicion of her husband's behaviour she told him to leave, putting his clothes in a bundle outside the door. 'He told her, "I am not going anywhere!" and refused to leave. It is very difficult for a wife to drive her husband from the house'.[20] When male clients are known to be HIV positive and disclose that they are having unprotected sexual relations, persuasion rather than exposure is the practice. They do not pursue men who have abandoned their children and left wives or partners infected. They avoid a language of confrontation in gender relations, instead emphasising reconciliation and mutual understanding. Of one client, Kaijage (1993: 272) says: 'She had to come to terms with her anger at her husband's family for rejecting her at a time when she felt they needed each other most. She has learned better ways of persuading him to do things rather than blaming him, and he is no longer reacting in an angry defensive way'.

That women are angry about men's behaviour – and that many of WAMATA's female clients/members feel themselves powerless, is undeniable. They are not simply seeking 'information' but influential allies in their real and lonely struggles with men. At a women's group meeting observed in July 1998, this seemed very evident. Ostensibly the women were learning about the female condom:

A demonstrator showed pictures illustrating how to wear these condoms – you have to put it in like a diaphragm from a squatting position... She demonstrated using her handbag as stand-in for the womb, showing how you pushed it in as far as it would go with your finger – 'it is very long'. The audience was shown samples of condoms, and invited to ask questions. Questions followed, about possible dangers – of leaving it in for a long time, of whether it could be 'lost inside', whether its rings might not cause pain. However, then there was an interesting exchange: 'Can a man tell if you are wearing it? I mean can you use it without him knowing that you have it in?'. [The woman facilitating the meeting responds]: 'No, you should discuss it with him. He can tell you have it on and he may need help to guide his thing in the right place'. A young woman interrupts: 'Sometimes women don't want sex at all, but men want it all the time!'. The facilitator responded to this firstly by explaining why women might not want sex – the aftermath of male brutality or lack of knowledge: 'Our men don't know 'romance' (she used the English word) – they can rush in when you are in the middle of household tasks and expect you to be ready. We are like cars – can they go if their engines have no oil or grease?'[21]

The inclusive 'we' connotes appeal to an essential women's experiential knowledge, whilst at the same time the notion of 'romance' puts her vision beyond most of the experience of the audience. For them the reality is, 'Men may force you when you are asleep and not ready!' or, 'I know of one girl who was raped when she was 13 and now she can't have sex without screaming and yelling with fear'. The facilitator responds that 'this girl needs urgent psychiatric help'.

Women members demand that WAMATA address men. 'They suggested that we should be holding more seminars for men because women are sensitised enough'.[22] 'Women felt that they had no power to protect themselves from getting HIV infection, they felt that the prevention strategies were protecting men more than women'.[23] Staff say that the bid to extend campaigning to men 'came from women themselves. They say: "We know these things, please help us to make our men know"'. Both WAMATA and SWAAT have moved towards targeting men for inclusion.[24] Attempts to do this have not always been productive. Working with mixed groups sometimes silences the women or leads to polarised debate.

Finally, there are distinctive ways in which gendered norms are transgressed in the context of AIDS activism. The AIDS organisation constitutes an arena within which women may pursue class objectives more normally monopolised by men. In doing so they break some of the rules of how women should behave in the public arena. They assume an authority, which is dissonant with their social position, by demonstrating competence and expertise and wielding the power to give or withhold specialised knowledge. This may be asserted vis à vis men or, more commonly, against older women who would normally take precedence.

For women to display knowledge of sex and sexual matters in public can itself be transgressive and morally charged. Speaking openly of sex has always been taboo – it was a private and secret matter voiced only by those without self-respect or shame. Both men and women adhered to this view, though women were also expected to exhibit modesty and ignorance in such matters. AIDS has disrupted this discourse – and necessarily so. Women who become AIDS activists must overcome greater hostility in their public work, and they require great courage to speak openly. One example illustrates both the transgressive nature of AIDS work and its upturning of established rules of gender relations:

> A WAMATA worker related how she had been leaving the office one day and encountered some men repairing a house nearby. They accosted her at first with banter, almost certainly intended to embarrass and humiliate her: 'Oh, why don't you show us some condoms!' She did not turn a hair, but went back and got some condoms from the office and showed them to the men. 'Yes we see, mama – but *how* do you put them on?!' Again she was unperturbed and went and fetched the penis mould and brought it out and showed them how to correctly fit on a condom.[25]

She added that the mood then changed – whereas at first they were all jeering, it ended up as a very serious discussion. When some asked questions that sounded disrespectful, the others rebuked them.

AIDS organisations can thus be seen as an arena in which new modes of interaction between men and women are being tried out, albeit these can only be fully understood in terms of cross-cutting divisions of class and generation.

Conclusions

At the same time that AIDS activism is confronting the AIDS epidemic – and in the case of WAMATA it has made some innovative and remarkable advances in this endeavour – other struggles are proceeding which deserve analysis. AIDS is a disease transmitted largely through sexual relations – inevitably, then, it raises questions about the existing pattern of gender relations. These questions relate not only to the greater vulnerability of women in situations of gender inequity. The organisation itself becomes a setting in which gender struggles are played out – over women's right to speak openly on sexual matters, even where this transgresses gendered norms, for women to assert equality with male colleagues and to consolidate their class position through processes of professionalisation and so on.

In a context of economic impoverishment and state withdrawal from public service provision, it is not surprising that class fractions exiled from state employment find a home in AIDS work (amongst other voluntary sector activities). The threat of epidemic infection to all, irrespective of class, gives them a potent incentive to prophylactic action. Conversely, involvement in AIDS work risks moral and social contamination. It breaches the social distance which class cultures build between unequals. In confronting poverty-stricken fellow-sufferers who devise their own instrumental modes of class survival in their relations with AIDS organisations, petty-bourgeois AIDS activists develop forms of interaction, which whilst genuinely sharing knowledge, may also symbolically mark their class difference. Class projects of rescue and uplift are pronounced.

Were it not for foreign donors these class projects could not easily proceed. We cannot ignore the impact that international agencies have had on the objectives and modes of operation of AIDS organisations. Effectively they dictate the terms, however benevolent. Kaijage (1995:199) argues that, 'although they choose to bypass governments, Northern funding sources demand the same type of bureaucratic structures from grassroots NGOs. The result is that NGOs in developing countries are competing for scant resources, yet a high demand is placed on them in terms of managerial ability, financial accountability and proposal writing'. Donors also require them to fill a welfare gap cheaply and shape their modes of doing this.

Whilst beholden to foreign donors for their very existence, it would be unduly cynical to see AIDS organisations as merely a response to 'the changing complexion of the international aid agenda' which local people have learnt to 'exploit' (Chabal and Daloz, 1999: 23). There is nothing inevitable about success in funding bids – it is a constant struggle. The existence of indigenous AIDS associations, adapting meagre resources to the tragic circumstances of AIDS in Tanzania, continues *despite* the conditionality of funding and its potential as stranglehold. If such associations are barely evidence of an autonomous and independent civil society, free from state control,[26] they cannot be dismissed as merely opportunistic. In a setting of risk to all parties, they represent an exciting maelstrom of ideas and practices, where struggle on many levels – class, gender, generation, as well as against AIDS – is generating innovative ideas, novel forms of activity and path-breaking new relations. We can learn so much.

Notes

1 In full: *Walio katika Mapambano ya AIDS, Tanzania* (Those in the struggle against AIDS in Tanzania).

2 This chapter is based on the authors' observation of AIDS organisations and interviews with AIDS activists in Dar es Salaam, 1995–99. It also draws on field studies of the impact of AIDS on gender relations in Dar es Salaam by members of our research team: Japhet Lutimba, Scholastica Mokake, Julius Mwabuki, Feddy Mwanga and Zubeida Tumbo-Masabo, several of whom were also either officers or volunteers in WAMATA, WAMATA Youth or SWAAT. Additional work was carried out by Marjorie Mbilinyi and Julius Mwabuki through a survey of AIDS NGOs in Dar es Salaam (1996). Janet Bujra takes responsibility for the theoretical framing of this piece, noting that it evolved out of stimulating encounters with AIDS activists and lively debate within our research group.

3 NGOs come in many guises. Here we focus on indigenous non-state welfare organisations operating at the national level. The scale of such enterprises distinguishes

them from small community-based associations. Within organisations such as WAMATA we distinguish paid staff (referred to as AIDS 'workers' or 'activists') from those whom they assist – though the boundary is permeable and nomenclature is contested.

4 We use the term class in a relational sense here, not as an indexical device to distinguish between people of different income levels.

5 It ranked second in cumulative AIDS cases. These statistics cannot be taken as more than suggestive. In 1998, the reported number of AIDS cases in Tanzania was only 109,863, whilst the estimated total was 549,315 (NACP, 1999: 6). HIV prevalence is measured via women attending 'sentinel sites' in ante-natal clinics, or through the testing of donated blood. By 1995, sentinel sites had been established in eleven out of twenty regions, but only twelve sites in five regions reported back. By 1998, this was ten out of two (NACP, 1996, 1999). Blood donations come disproportionately from younger fitter men, and the facilities for collecting and testing are sometimes inadequate.

6 During the 1980s when the last census was held (Government of Tanzania, 1988), Dar es Salaam had an annual average growth rate of 4.8 per cent (compared with the overall national rate of 2.8 per cent).

7 Fieldworkers' report on Manzese, Dar es Salaam (J. Lutimba and J. Mwabuki, 1997). Adapted slightly to make clear sense.

8 S. Mokake, field report from Kigamboni, Dar es Salaam, 1995. Men are reluctant to use condoms in encounters with sex workers, even though this is cheaper (Sh.500 was quoted in one report). Sex without a condom may vary from twice to ten times as much, depending on the woman's desirability. Women who agree augment their income, but put their lives at risk – as do their customers (Mokake, field report on Kigamboni, 1997; J. Mwabuki reporting on prostitutes buying condoms from a shop in Kinondoni, August 1998).

9 Kaijage has written about the formation of WAMATA and about the issues it faces (Kaijage, 1991, 1993, 1995). She is hereinafter refereed to as 'Mama Theresa', the normal term of respect.

10 Quotations, unless otherwise attributed, come from interviews with paid worker activists. To protect confidentiality, they have been deliberately anonymised.

11 Amongst others, the World Food Programme, the World Health Organisation, the Humanistic Institute for International Cooperaton (HIVOS), the Southern African Training Programme (SAT), the Danish Association for International Cooperation (MS), the Social Action Trust Fund (SATF) and Terre des Hommes (TDH).

12 J. Bujra, fieldnotes, 22 May 1995.

13 *Shangazi* is the Swahili term for 'father's sister' or paternal aunt.

14 F. Mwanga, fieldnotes, 1998: 22.

15 Z. Tumbo-Masabo, field report, 1995.

16 S. Mokake, field report, 1995: 6.

17 Not all clients are poor. Kaijage (1993: 272) refers to one with a good job who needed emotional rather than material support, whilst teachers and secretaries are noted below. However, over time, the association of AIDS organisations with the materially destitute and with social exposure has led the better-off to shun them. A worker at SWAAT said: 'ministers, big people, they wouldn't come – they would have other ways of getting medicines'. In another case reported, where the daughter of a prominent family was dying, the 'shame' was hidden from everyone. Her father secured all the drugs he could afford – AZT, Kemron etc. Their side effects rendered the girl deaf, blind, and unable to eat. She died quickly, deprived of the social and psychological support which organisations like WAMATA provide.

18 J. Lutimba and J. Mwabuki, field report, 1998.

19 Bond and Vincent (1997: 103) report similar attitudes in a study of AIDS activism amongst students in Uganda.

20   J. Bujra, fieldnotes, May 1995.
21   J. Bujra, fieldnotes, July 1998.
22   S. Mokake, fieldnotes, 1996: 12.
23   S. Mokake, fieldnotes, 1996: 8.
24   F. Mwanga, fieldnotes, 1998: 13.
25   J. Bujra, fieldnotes, 26 May 1995.
26   Whilst state surveillance has always been an element in the operation of NGOs in Tanzania, public recognition of AIDS work has been lacking until recently. Political leaders now publicly acknowledge the crisis posed by AIDS.

9   The struggle continues: some conclusions

Carolyn Baylies and Janet Bujra

The scale and depth of the AIDS crisis has prompted calls to enlist women's organising capacities and collective energy in campaigns for protection. Women have been targeted partly because they themselves have lined up to assist as primary carers within families, through religious groups offering compassion to those who are sick or bereaved, via informal networks providing mutual support around rites of passage, and through more formal charitable and service organisations, NGOs and community-based organisations. While men are also involved in such activities, their numbers are dwarfed by women fulfilling roles as carers, volunteers and educators, whether in the domestic sphere or the informal and formal sectors of the public sphere.

Women's community care activities are generally tolerated, even applauded, unless the time supporting others is perceived to encroach on the care and sustenance of their immediate families. However, women's success in mounting campaigns of protection can immediately encounter the same intransigent beliefs and practices which contribute to their vulnerability to HIV. Women's accumulated experience in networking, combined with their first hand knowledge of how gender relations make them susceptible to risk of infection, put them in a position not just to 'speak the truth' but to organise around campaigns of protection. Yet doing so generates resistance, given those same gender relations which place them in a disadvantaged position both within the context of intimate relations and within the wider society.

The idea of gender as a relational concept is not usually understood by AIDS practitioners. For policy review and planning, 'sex' is employed as a variable, with acknowledgement of categorical differences between men and women (in rates of prevalence or use of condoms). However, these differences are less often understood as a function of the way men and women relate to each other. The new conceptual language of 'gender' has been widely interpreted to mean special programmes for women. Where men appear they do so in deviant sexual guise – as promiscuous truckers, soldiers, sugar daddies – in much in the same way that sex workers predominate in accounts of women and AIDS. The generality of ordinary men do not appear, and there is little acknowledgement that it is in 'normal' social relations between the sexes that danger lies. It is not gendered difference but gendered inequality that puts both women and men at risk.

Changing constructions of sexuality

Understanding the ways in which sexuality is constructed and gender relations configured is crucial for strategies of protection against HIV. The subordination of women's needs and desires in relations of intimacy came through in all of our case studies, expressed in a variety of ways. Understandings of sexuality and the content of sexual practice are embedded in specific cultural histories and are the products of particular experiences of social and economic change. As they evolve, such understandings apply differently to those in different social locations defined by age and marital status, as well as gender (and other social variables). They form the backdrop through which AIDS is experienced and its ramifications felt. However, the epidemic in its turn has influenced the ongoing construction and reconstruction of sexuality and the beliefs and behaviours which constitute it.

Accounts of Kapulanga, Rungwe and Kanyama focused on this broader context, attempting to make sense of the response to AIDS and the way blame has been cast particularly on women and young people. In Kapulanga interpretations of affliction based on taboos associated with women's physiology were drawn on in attempts to come to terms with AIDS. Analysis of the situation in Rungwe showed how disquiet about women's greater economic independence has influenced perceptions about AIDS. In that case older people often directed their anger at women traders and the young for abandoning former practices and embodying new materialistic values: 'the girls are hungry for money and have no desire to follow the old traditions'. In Kanyama and Kapulanga, earlier interpretations of certain illnesses as resulting from sexual transgressions have also been invoked in attempts to explain AIDS and distinguish it (or not) as a new illness.

In North America and Europe, dominant reactions to AIDS fed on deep seated anxiety about changing patterns of sexual behaviour and what some considered to be an aberrant form of sexuality. From this perspective, AIDS has represented retribution for moral transgression (Patton, 1985; Alcorn, 1988; Weeks, 1988, 1993). In Africa, with heterosexual transmission predominant, it has not been sexual orientation which is at issue, but promiscuity – both real and imagined.[1] While this critique has occasionally depicted men as culpable (for example, sugar daddies or rich men), it has equally, if not more strenuously, condemned female sex workers or women regarded as not 'respecting themselves'. But masculinity – and the behaviour associated with it – has seldom been a concern within public discourse, even though its specific importance was identified early on by a number of commentators (Ankrah, 1991; de Bruyn, 1992; Obbo, 1993; Heise and Elias, 1995). Advocacy of partner reduction has been qualified by an assumption that men's multiple partnering cannot be expected to be eliminated altogether and needs to be coupled with much stronger advice to use condoms. And here the implicit message has been that condoms are appropriate for casual encounters, but not for marriage.

Box 9.1 Rural men respond to AIDS

Interviews with two men in 1996, both Muslims from rural Lushoto, indicate a distinctive contrast in responses to AIDS, which reflect both generational and experiential differences. Jamal is a young man whose sister died of AIDS. Most unusually he cared for her intimately until her death. He is aware of the dilemmas facing young people and of the need to use condoms. Mzee Mganga is a traditional healer, a much older man, whose occupation has involved him in treatment of the opportunistic infections of AIDS. His moral diagnosis of its spread and his punitive attitude towards women and those who use condoms is in marked contrast to that of Jamal.

Jamal

Jamal is aged 29 and was educated to primary grade 4. He became a middleman selling crops in Arusha and lived there for several years. He still looked smart and possessed an umbrella but his house was shabby, and he was struggling to make ends meet. However, he still had two small pieces of land, one inherited and one bought. His sister's illness had taken all his savings and 'I have fallen far. I am just at home now, working for others as an agricultural labourer'.

'As far as AIDS is concerned, my sister died of it right here – she was a trader in Muheza and she met someone who gave it to her. We went to the hospitals in Lushoto and Bumbuli and to traditional healers. When we took her to the healer he cut her to rub in some medicines and then he cut someone else with that same razor blade – but they are still healthy.

In Bumbuli they tried to hide it from me, but in Lushoto they told me not to waste any more money as she had children who would need care when she died. We buried her here. She had diarrhoea and vomiting and then she got very weak. All her bones stuck out and her flesh disappeared. It went on for 2 or 3 years. In the end there were maggots coming out when she had diarrhoea. I cared for her because my mother was dead. (Other relatives told me that his mother committed suicide on discovering her daughter was dying of AIDS.)

This is a disease that you don't get right here – it's from outside. A man might return from those places (Dar etc.) and infect two or three girls. Then young men in the village might sleep with them thinking they have never been anywhere – they don't realise – and that's the way it is spread. If young people use condoms then they don't get it. I used to use them when I was in Arusha doing business. Of course married people are unsafe too. A wife might be given money to go to the market and there she is offered money or gifts by a man to do sex – the husband hasn't any idea, he sleeps with her as usual... Married people need to discuss and be concerned and protect themselves. Some use condoms for protection, or to space births, or because they are afraid of each other. Not that a wife can demand this – unless you have been away and she is shocked at your appearance when you return, or you start to get very thin. Using condoms makes more sense than abstaining from sex. When my sons get bigger I will tell them they need to protect themselves, especially from casual sex, and they should use condoms, and carry condoms. I will leave Mama to tell the girls'.

Mzee Mganga

This man, aged 50, is a successful healer with three wives and land. He has been married twelve times and has twelve children. He has a licence to practice healing from the government and goes back and forth to Dar es Salaam and Tanga to treat people – at the time he was interviewed he had just been called to Dar es Salaam to treat a women who was paralysed down one side and he was preparing medicines to take with him.

Mzee Mganga never went to school – 'in those days my head was poor and I couldn't take things in'. As a young man he had worked for 5 years in Tanga as a cook for Europeans. He became a healer after he was himself struck low with a bad back and he was visited by a ghost who told him how to get better and how to cure others.

He began to hear about AIDS when people came to him with the disease and he couldn't cure them. He would give them injections, but 'they die and there is no real help – I tell them to go to hospital. Now I can tell if they have AIDS – I have a test'. The 'HIV test' entailed mixing together the saliva and blood of the sick person: 'if he has the disease then it smells foul'.

'The symptoms are diarrhoea and vomiting with headache and severe wasting. It comes from adultery, immoral sex. It spreads more in the big towns because of women who are looking for sex – young girls too, unmarried – it's business. Here married people are in trouble if they go after 'outside wives', and husbands are warning their wives these days. As for young people, they should be more concerned about their drinking and fornication. A drunkard has no thought for AIDS, marijuana smokers don't care. Condoms don't help – the "water" drips out and blood could get into open wounds. A wife who asks you to use those things is not a wife but a prostitute. Some wives are not satisfied. If she asked, you would guess and accuse her of going with someone else! However, men who have outside partners should protect their wives by using condoms with them.

A woman who is lacking in the proper respect can deceive you – she can say she is going to a "meeting" and it is not a meeting at all. You have the right to refuse her. You don't beat her – the lawful way is to warn her or divorce her, rather than hit her.

The only men who would refuse to have sex with their wives are homosexuals (*wahanithi*). I have treated some of them with roots to change their ways.

These days people break customary rules and talk openly about sex – they talk rubbish even in front of mothers now. You don't need to be taught about sex – at a certain age you just know. It's God's doing...- When I was young you used to be treated with medicines so that you were unable to behave badly, run after women. The medicine "imprisoned" you. The idea of giving young people condoms is shocking – to begin with they are not much use anyway, but also the one who presses for those things is a dirty type – you can't ask your father for such things – he will respond "you savage!".

Yes, the children of those who are infected will die, and you must make arrangements for the children who will be left behind. I treated one woman in Mlalo – she had no husband. She had come back from Tanga with her child and both of them were infected. I told her to go to her home and not to waste any more money on healers or hospitals, but she didn't listen. Both she and the child died. It's better to test before you have children'.

Despite recent literature unravelling essentialist views of 'masculinity' (and insisting instead on the plurality of 'masculinities'),[2] it is as a powerful hegemonic force that women encounter masculinity in sexual relations. The very hegemony of masculine definitions of sexual behaviour has become constructed as a problem for women to contend with, but not for men to confront. Although the specifics may differ, the reality for women in African societies has global resonance. It is in terms of men's pleasure and under men's control that the sexual act primarily occurs, and women, young and old, married and unmarried, often feel they have little say in sexual relations. This is hegemony imbued with power and posing an often palpable threat, as evident from the phraseology which women often use: 'what can you do'?;[3] 'you do not dare';[4] or, even more emphatically, 'that is the "law" of marriage. That is what constitutes marriage. You can't say no'.[5] Power applies most strikingly in coercive sex, as experienced by former members of the Maisha group in Lushoto in the form of rape, but is also implied by the comments of the Muchinka drama women that requesting a partner to use condoms can lead to violence within a marriage,[6] and the remark of a young woman in a focus group in Kanyama that 'a man cannot leave a girl alone; they always pester a girl until she agrees'.[7]

Women sometimes question the extent and rigidity of such power, indicating an ongoing process of struggle and of some change. In response to the suggestion that women are forced into submission by constant harassment, for example, another of the group's participants replied sharply: 'if you agree it means you also want. If you don't want there is no way he can force you'[8]. This suggests that women's acquiescence to prevailing norms is a factor serving to perpetuate them, but also that resistance is possible. Many women are unpersuaded and have the scars to show for it. The very pervasiveness of notions about male control in sexual encounters speak of how firmly they are grounded in everyday life and how the terms of women's existence often leave little room for anything but compliance, even if covert means and strategies may be adopted to gain manoeuvrability within close personal relationships.

Economic dependence and gendered power relations

This subordination of women in relations of intimacy is paralleled by and intrinsically linked to their disadvantaged position within the wider society, as evident in their lesser access to education and training and less frequent occupancy of positions of public authority. But the broader structure of gender bias is particularly epitomised by women's economic position. Women's limited education, lack of saleable skills and generally disadvantaged position within the labour market often implies economic dependence on men – either as husbands, gatekeepers to economic activities or direct purchasers of their sexual services – contributing to and reinforcing their restricted power within sexual encounters. The specific nature of the link between social location and leverage within intimate relations varies. But in its different guises it came up again and again.

Women attempting to gain an independent income have often been condemned, particularly when engaging in trade and especially when having to travel in connection with their business. Older men in Mansa spoke heatedly about market women: 'especially women who go to buy fish for sale, they infect their husbands' and insisted that they would not allow their own wives to engage in business which required their moving from one town to another.[9] In Rungwe it was alleged that 'these women traders go out of husband's and relatives' control – it is easy to conduct love affairs'. In Lushoto, anxiety and condemnation in equal measure were expressed about young women running off to town to seek work. While often tinged with a degree of hysteria and invalid in its blanket stereotyping of women operating in the market economy, it is true that sexual liaisons may accompany trade. This sometimes reflects patterns of male power, with access to key goods or market opportunities dependent on an exchange of sexual favours (Mushingeh *et al.*, 1990–91). But as one woman conceded in a focus group discussion in Kanyama: 'Some women would like to start a business. If there is no man to support her, she will go for other ways of getting the money. Through that she will be infected'.[10]

Those who engage directly in sex work are seen as most reprehensible. Blatantly transgressing the sexual roles prescribed for women, their activity is a necessary adjunct to the masculine norm of greater sexual mobility. These are the women, in the parlance of others, who do not respect themselves, who frequent bars and who are sometimes suspected of being carriers of HIV, with greater capacity to escape its impact than those who are 'morally upright'[11]. Such views are frequently softened by an understanding of the pressures compelling young women toward sex work. If not condoning their behaviour, many accept it as an outcome of factors beyond their control. Such women may even be regarded as emblematic of the way in which poverty – and sometimes the impact of SAPs – is directly linked to the spread of AIDS. As a traditional healer in Kanyama asserted: 'they have to earn a living somehow. For instance, a man would come to you and offer K3,000 (about US $3). Tomorrow, he comes back with K5,000 (about US $5). You cannot refuse. The bottom line is poverty'.[12]

Sex work is a fluid category and the exchange of sex for material goods may take more informal forms, associated with boyfriends or casual liaisons. In some cases these too are the outcomes of economic need. A woman in Mansa explained that 'if you don't have food you can go to another man hoping to get some money for food'.[13] A similar point was made by a woman in Kapulanga: 'if we find someone ready to give us something, we will accept the money, provide what he needs and then feed our children. Do you expect us to sit down and watch our children go hungry day after day because we should abstain from sex? No!' (quoted in Sikwibele, 1996).

Not all are willing to countenance even the hunger of children as rationale for selling sex, nor to accept that this as justification for what they regard as fundamentally immoral behaviour. Yet it is *women's* dire need which can put them at particular risk of HIV, highlighting the way that economic position is bound up with gender relations. Young girls' lack of skills or alternative economic opportunities may lead them to sell sex, while boys, similarly affected by poverty, are less likely to adopt such a strategy, and if they do, this is scarcely acknowledged.

Increasing awareness of the gender aspects of AIDS

Excerpts from focus discussions conducted across the six sites provide clear evidence of increasing awareness, not just of the particular vulnerability of women, but of the fact that this is grounded in economic considerations, gender relations and specifically in men's behaviour. This grassroots insight accords with growing acknowledgement from official sectors about deficits in women's claim on human rights, cultures of gendered oppression and the way economic relations impede women's ability to protect themselves against HIV.

There is also evidence of a process of collective learning at community level and of attempts to address behaviours putting both men and women at risk. The AIDS epidemic has brought sexual behaviour into the realm of public discourse in a way unimaginable a decade earlier and has led to debate and reflection on practices deemed harmful, or at the least unhelpful, in the face of HIV. Thus, in Zambia there has been official condemnation of sexual forms of 'cleansing' following the death of a spouse, of the grabbing of property from widows, and of the practice of dry sex. While none of these practices has been fully eliminated, they have at least been held up to scrutiny. In parts of Tanzania men are openly questioning indigenous customs such as wife inheritance, noting examples where this practice had led to a trail of fatalities. It needs emphasising, however, that men have more power to reject such customs than women; indeed women may suffer if as elderly wives they have no male protector or provider.

Effectiveness of collective initiatives

On the ground, there is a thirst for more detailed knowledge. People frequently asked members of the research teams for information and 'seminars'. They were impatient when it seemed that we were coming to elicit their views rather than to provide knowledge about AIDS. It was not just facts they wanted, but much more. They wanted to know what they could do, how they could protect themselves, how they could be sure that their children would not be infected and would live to become parents and grandparents. We did answer questions, conduct seminars and liaise between groups and individuals who might provide them with more sustainable support, but we also persistently turned the question back to those we met, asking them what they thought was necessary to be done, what they felt they could do.

Most people on the ground were also convinced about the importance and validity of community-based collective action around AIDS. Affirmation of the need for community action represents the common destination of a number of different lines of argument. It reflects an appreciation that those in the locality have expertise, a stake in the longevity of their community and concern for their neighbours. It reflects a perceived need by governments to devolve to community level and to enlist as much participation as possible, given pressing need and limited resources. It reflects optimism by some development theorists and practitioners in the possibility of grass-roots participation leading to greater accountability and ultimately to greater democracy.

Strategies aimed at the 'community' must themselves be held up to scrutiny, however, particularly where they fail to acknowledge divisions and conflicting interests within communities. Such divisions have been most graphically illustrated here in the Lushoto case. These very divisions, along lines of gender or age or power, are implicated in the spread of AIDS. Interrogating the nature of these divisions may lead to strategies which locate vulnerability to AIDS in broader structures of inequality and human rights deficits. It may also foster collective action by local groups of people who are particularly at risk, be they married women or adolescent females or sex workers. Placing the initiative with those whose vulnerability is greater, while drawing on their experience and knowledge, may contribute to a more public exposure of inequalities and provide impetus towards their reversal. However, disadvantaged groups cannot play this role without support and resources.

This brings us back to our starting point, of investigating the potential of women's groups in campaigns of protection against HIV. An evaluation of their potential effectiveness can be carried at out several levels – the objectives they set for themselves, their impact on the lives of their members and the contribution they may make to broader transformations identified as crucial for fighting the AIDS epidemic, not least in respect of gender relations.

Meeting group objectives

Some forms of collective activity are primarily geared to the needs of group members. This applies, for example, to income generating or skills training projects directed at those whose lack of economic security is considered to put them at particular risk of HIV infection. In such cases success depends on whether skills are acquired or income generated. However, many groups are engaged in outreach activities, whether in prevention or care or a combination of these. The effectiveness of such activities necessarily varies with the specific nature of the work, and may not be susceptible to precise measurement.

Organisations are increasingly disciplined by funders to monitor their performance and to count up their achievements. This applies not only to national organisations like WAMATA, but even the smallest village groups granted small sums to further their activities. Evaluation generally proceeds on the basis of what can be quantified – the number of home visits made, condoms distributed, performances given, or size of audiences addressed.[14] But achievements are not always easily quantifiable, nor are those which are quantifiable always the most fundamental. Particularly problematic is demonstrating a causal link between group activities and wider changes in behaviour (Hughes-d'Aeth, 1998), not least because impact studies require more sophisticated techniques than many on the ground have access to and need to be grounded in base-line assessment.

While effectiveness may be confined to a specific timeframe in the eyes of funders, and indeed to a specified budget, collective endeavour at community level is not limited to project work, and both its sustainability, and evolution of the form and content of specific initiatives are particularly important in a context where need not only continues, but escalates. An initial flush of enthusiasm, infused with good will and expectation of benefits, makes subsequent disappointment all the more crushing when efforts fail and the activity slips away as occurred in Kanyama; or (as in the case of Maisha in Lushoto and the Natweshe Club in Mansa), its focus shifts away from the original objectives or target group. Such outcomes are particularly worrying, not just because an initial investment in time and training seems virtually wasted, but because disillusionment can turn to apathy, undermining the potential for regeneration or reconsolidation of efforts.

Groups have their own trajectories which vary in terms of initial objectives, resources, and local circumstances, so that generalisations may be hazardous. Yet from the various case studies reported here, some general points can be made. Much rests on organisational form – the way a group is structured and the way in which the attributes and interests of its members and the nature of their activities accord with both immediate and longer-term objectives. Clarity of purpose, feasibility of objectives and collective agreement about the nature and importance of objectives are prerequisites for effectiveness. A degree of homogeneity of membership, along lines of age or marital status may also be important, not least as these may imply commonality of background and outlook and limit divisive differences. Many groups collapse through failures of leadership, as we have seen. Charismatic founders die or move on, having made themselves indispensable; leadership may be lacking and the group uncoordinated; or systems of democratic accountability between members and those they serve remain undeveloped. To the extent that members share a common commitment, however, and, more importantly, exhibit a shared sense of responsibility to the group and its work, the greater may be its effectiveness. When collective learning occurs via collective reflection on activities, groups may be energised.

Personal costs and benefits

Two dimensions may be particularly important in assessing groups – the relationship between personal commitment, individual cost and personal benefit, and that between organisational objectives and available resources.[15] As indicated by negative outcomes, where individuals drop out because benefit has declined, or is too low, or does not match their expectations, individual calculation of the balance between cost and benefit is crucial. This may apply at all levels. As Hughs-d'Aeth (1998) notes in an evaluation of several of the larger AIDS NGOs in Zambia, under-staffing often results when remuneration is inadequate to attract and retain good quality professionals to co-ordinate programmes. Adequate remuneration is equally, perhaps more, important at community level, but here the tension between voluntarism on the one hand and compensation for personal costs accrued on the other is also particularly acute. The call for voluntarism (though legitimate) can be particularly galling when made by those enjoying the comfort of salaried and high-status posts. AIDS activity as a business both breeds and reflects class inequalities, as has been noted in the account of WAMATA, and can induce competition for the rewards perceived to be available, as well as resentment among those less successful in obtaining them. It is important to recognise how such dynamics of inequality permeate AIDS work.

AIDS generates a community response and a desire in many quarters to do something for those whose suffering is greatest. As much as it undermines families and communities, causing division and recrimination, it also engenders a spirit of altruism and collective concern. Governments and aid agencies design their policies to encourage these altruistic tendencies; they are crucial to any strategy of containment and care. However, there are limits to how much those in communities most in need can give freely of their time and material resources. Questions need to be raised about how costs are apportioned within a community and how compensation should in turn be distributed to ensure that existing inequalities along gender and other lines are not entrenched through the very process of work on behalf of the community. Benefits are not all material, but material situation is a crucial foundation for offering the energy and time which collective activities require.

Organisational objectives and resources

Local groups often concluded that the crisis brought by AIDS stretched existing resources so far that even their minimal objectives could only be met with difficulty. Though rich in personal skills, they were rarely endowed with material resources sufficient to compensate either for their time and personal reserves, or wider costs to the community associated with disrupted production or lost income following from illness and death. Nor did they always possess the skills required to sustain their organisation, offer care and support and provide appropriate and effective educational messages. Need for external resources and a broader collective responsibility, extending to local and national governments, and beyond to institutions and agencies at a global level, is now accepted and articulated with an increasing sense of urgency.[16] Yet the amount on offer is far, far less than required, with a fifteen fold increase needed to make good the deficit at the turn of the century (when official assistance for HIV/AIDS in Africa stood at some US $160 million against an estimated need of as much as US $2.3 billion).[17]

It is not just the amount, however, but the form in which assistance is extended which is at issue. Appropriate support needs to be negotiated through joint consultation. Rather than have agendas dictated to them, groups need to set agendas for themselves. While accountability to donors is necessary, they also need to be accountable to their own members and those they assist. They need useful and readily available advice. They need training and encouragement. If they are to extend innovative working and expand services of prevention and care, they need genuine collaboration with partners – whether government or 'global' – who are reliable and efficient, who keep their promises and share their knowledge.

Here, as elsewhere in AIDS work, the objectives of increasing knowledge, self reliance, shared responsibility and greater equity need to be applied to the means through which 'assistance' is proffered. Donors and international NGOs often wish to promote a local sense of ownership and often profess an appreciation of indigenous knowledge and local experience. Yet their methods can be condescending, reconstructing lines of dependence. Their message can be confused and contradictory, breeding a desperate attempt by those on the ground to 'figure out' what is wanted, what new device is required – be it an 'action plan', a 'mission statement' or an 'internal audit'. Donors' generosity may be fickle, with funds and other assistance extended for a while and then withdrawn, without means of local sustainability having been nurtured and with need even greater than before.

When it is government from whom local people anticipate support (whether direct, or as an opening to foreign donors) then here too they may have to put on an appropriate show. We have occasionally observed travesties of AIDS work, when women's groups are called and paid to perform for visiting dignitaries. Local officials may need evidence that they are taking the issue of AIDS seriously; desperately poor people are ready with song and dance routines to put food in their children's mouths. However, if AIDS prevention is furthered in this way, it is purely incidental.

Those on the receiving end of external assistance are generally grateful at one level but often deeply critical at another. They are aware that their objectives can be distorted by external agendas and rules of engagement. They are demoralised when support or recognition fails to materialise. Both external agents and local actors are engaged in a learning process, with some changes having occurred on both sides. The essential inequalities between giver and receiver may be impossible to overcome, but it is important that they are brought into the open and jointly reflected upon.

Empowering potential of collective action?

Collective action at the local level is a crucial resource in AIDS work, providing support and care to those in need and extending messages of protection. How far does it also have an impact on participants, increasing their awareness and strengthening their ability to make changes in their own lives? How far is it also a means to empowerment? The notion of empowerment is ambiguous, insofar as its boundaries are diffuse and its level of application unspecified. Reference is often made not just to individual empowerment, but also to collective empowerment with implications for the organisation or for the social group from which its members are drawn (Young, 1993; Kabeer, 1994; Rowlands, 1997).

Individual empowerment is typically treated as equivalent to increased self-confidence or sense of self-efficacy, combining a psychological state with increased knowledge and skills. This is important in its own right, particularly when relations of subordination systematically undermine self-esteem and induce doubts about personal capabilities. Self-belief and the confidence to act upon it, to speak of the truth that one has experienced, are crucial to both personal development and the ability to share talents and strengths.

In our case studies there were many who testified to the personal benefits they gained from collective initiatives, often framed as increased knowledge or increased skills. In Lushoto, the girls in Maisha learned some basic sewing skills and the celebration which inaugurated the group brought them, if only briefly, a degree of public respect. The women in Lisach in Mansa acquired important skills through their craft activities. Members of the Muchinka drama group spoke repeatedly of their increased knowledge about AIDS. Across all the groups many had gained the confidence and ability to tell others about AIDS. Christian traditional educators had incorporated AIDS messages in their work. A mother of one of the girls in Maisha affirmed that her daughter's involvement had opened up the issue so that she herself could discuss the dangers of HIV with her other children. Women counselled their older children to take HIV tests and told their young ones not to pick up used condoms.

But was there any deeper impact? How far is knowledge put into personal practice? That knowledge is not always converted into protective behaviour, even by those who 'know best' is indicated by Reid's (n.d.) comment that 'those caught up in this pursuit (AIDS work) rarely use condoms themselves, neither the bureaucrats nor the activists'. Baggaley *et al.*'s (1996) study of HIV counsellors in Zambia similarly found that although all favoured the use of condoms for protection against the virus, only 27 per cent had ever used one. Moreover, while about half of the women counsellors worried about the behaviour of their partners, they felt unable to discuss this with them.

Examination of impact at this level is difficult and largely depends on what people report about their behaviour and the rationales they provide in respect of it. The limited data we have, however, suggests that the degree to which individuals attempted to apply their knowledge to their own lives varied with their personal circumstances, as did the level of success they encountered. Insofar as their economic situation is not so desperate that they are driven into risky situations, women who are older and/or who are on their own are more often able to ensure protection than younger women or those who are married. The same applies to sex workers. Cases were reported of resistance to cultural prescriptions or positive action in favour of one's own health, which were claimed to be directly linked to both the knowledge gained from group involvement and the solidarity which the group offered. Two women within the Muchinka drama group, for example, had refused to be sexually cleansed after their husbands died. Another member of the group, also a widow, declared 'what I teach is what I do'. Knowing that her husband could have had AIDS, she had decided to remain unmarried for 10 years. Now that the time was almost up, she said that if she thought about getting married again, she would go for a test and ask her intended husband to do the same. 'If he refuses, he is not interested in me', she said, and that would be that.[18] Within marriage some discussion was also beginning to take place and some changes occurring. In Lushoto, middle-aged *kidembwa* women at least rehearsed dialogues they might have with their husbands, trying out: 'use that condom, husband!' and 'better to be beaten than to die'.

Among the girls in Maisha, in contrast, there was less evidence that increased knowledge about HIV had led to increased capability to ensure personal protection. Indeed two had been raped. A third had suffered 'marriage by capture', but she had subsequently left the relationship. Perhaps her previous experience with Maisha and the knowledge gained thereby had given her strength to return to her parents on the grounds of her fear that 'he may infect me'.

Greater awareness, self confidence and psychological strength can be important outcomes of collective activity, but we regard empowerment as more than this. In signifying a challenge to existing patterns of dominance and subordination, it is most appropriately couched in terms of a change in power *relations*. This is critical in the case of AIDS, since it is in the nature of gendered power relations that vulnerability resides. Thus, a heightened sense of self-efficacy needs not just to undergird a public face and public behaviour, but also to be deployed in the arena of intimate relations.

Collective action on the part of women has been extolled (Young, 1993; Kabeer, 1994) as a means not just to articulate women's interests in respect of prevailing gender relations, but also as a basis from which women can begin, both individually and collectively, to challenge the power relations they confront, whether on the personal or public level. This is a process of struggle and individual success may not be forthcoming, not least since such challenge is likely to generate male resistance. What is important to note, however, is that impact on either personal or public level varies with the specific character of collective activity and more so with its specific objectives.

AIDS prevention work has a particular 'advantage' in this regard over other sorts of collective activity (e.g. income generating or micro-credit or health education more broadly) in that it can specifically reveal the interconnection between the 'personal' and the 'political'. What is distinctive about women's collective action around AIDS prevention is precisely its potential to address close personal relations directly. AIDS work thus is not just about acquiring knowledge or learning skills; it is also about those sexual practices and power relations between men and women which put women in jeopardy because of their relative subordination.

Linkage between organisational methodologies and broader transformations

The potential inherent in work around AIDS prevention is not always realised. There are many prevention messages which counsel accommodation to prevailing gender relations or manoeuvring for partial safety within them. Moreover, much prevention work involves telling *others* what they should do – adults telling young people to abstain, IEC specialists telling commercial sex workers to use condoms, or market women in Mansa telling their female audiences not to engage in sexual cleansing or allow their personal greed to encourage a daughter to go off with a 'rich' man. Prevention work can portray those spreading AIDS as hapless, irresponsible or ignorant, as abandoning tradition or as sinners, without revealing or critiquing the underlying gendered power relations, sometimes compounded by economic exploitation, which systematically put women at risk. But what is important is that it has the capacity to do so, particularly if carried out by those in positions of vulnerability. It is on this basis that it can serve as a means of women's 'emancipation', through exposing the way in which unequal gender relations are harmful and their transformation both life preserving and enabling of more just and equitable outcomes.

In contrast to the liberatory potential of women's work in the area of AIDS prevention, initiatives concentrating on care and support can reinforce gender expectations and the prevailing gender division of labour. On the ground, as noted, it is overwhelmingly women who are involved in community-based home care programmes and in charitable work carried out under the auspices of religious groups. They often gain important skills and a sense of personal satisfaction in the process (Blinkhoff *et al.*, 1999). The work they perform is invaluable. Yet as du Guerny and Sjöberg (1993) caution, the tendency to rely on women's energies in this area can perpetuate the existing gender division of labour and, by overextending women's energies, particularly if performed on a voluntary basis, can reduce the potential for collective action which challenges prevailing gender relations. Hence du Guerny and Sjöberg (1993) suggest an increased enlisting of men's and boys' energies in caring work and a redistribution of skills. At the very least the level of need demands a greater sharing of these support and caring activities, as noted in the fury of women in Rungwe over the extra care responsibilities thrust on them. In Lushoto, the subject of AIDS and who was to blame for it immediately brought up issues of the unequal loads of men and women in domestic and family labour. Questioning and introducing a change in the division of labour associated with care and nurturing may thus lend impetus to broader changes in gender relations.

Box 9.2 AIDS generates gender and generational struggles

The following account comes from the transcript of a village meeting held in rural Lushoto in 1996. A village group, consisting of six men and six women, had been set up to co-ordinate responses to AIDS. Despite two of the men here supporting the view that women are oppressed, it is Ali's voice which expresses the more common stance of men in this community.

Facilitator (pointing out the importance of parents talking to and supporting their children in these dangerous times of AIDS): 'These days – the men will forgive me – sometimes mothers find themselves having to take most of the responsibility...'

Uproar broke out, with a middle-aged man, Ali, saying: 'I don't agree with you – this is not true!' and a younger man, Jamal, 29, saying: 'What Mama says is absolutely right. Some women here – I am telling you, they get up in the morning from sleeping with their husbands and they go to fetch water and they struggle to the market to get their flour ground and they return carrying the flour-bin – and the man – let's say me, I come home in the evening and I am drunk. I say 'Serve me the *ugali* (maize porridge)!' and I eat. And mama tells me she has been to Mombo to buy maize and get it ground and she has carried it back on her head. As for you, the man, where have you been all the day – in the bar! Do you, the man, have a right to that *ugali*? However, you eat it! (The men laugh uncomfortably). It's only some of the women who experience this, not all of them, I'm not saying all men are like this. However, many leave everything to their wives. Out of five hundred men you will find only two that really concern themselves with affairs of the household'.

Ali (ignoring Jamal and addressing the facilitator): 'However, what you said about fathers, I cannot accept it. Women also contribute to the irresponsibility of young people. The greater proportion of people are brought up by their mothers. In the morning you get up and you wake your child and say, 'go to school' and then you go off – maybe to the farm or to cut grass for the cow, or whatever it is you have to do. And you come back later and you find – ah! the child has not gone to school! You ask why and the child says that mama sent him on a job, heavens knows where. Or she didn't wash the child's school clothes because there was no soap. And the days go by, and it gets to Saturday and only then she asks for Sh100 to buy a bar of soap. As a man you have so many things to attend to, and you rely on her to think of things like soap for washing...'

A middle-aged woman, Ernestina, now intervenes: 'To be honest, men don't think of things like that – they rely on you to feed the child, clothe it and do everything – it doesn't even enter their minds that there is a child to be fed or that there may be money owing at school – all dad does is say 'Fatuma, get up and go to school'...'.

Ali: 'Ah no!'.

Now women are supporting Ernestina, all of them nodding vigorously, with Jamal's support, whilst the men are bemused, uncertain and uncomfortable, not knowing how the conversation has taken this turn.

Ernestina: 'Please forgive me, but it's true, men don't think of the responsibilities of home and family unless you remind them'.

Ali: 'Not so!'.

Out of a babble of contending voices one now prevails convincingly and with quiet authority – Musa, an elderly man who is treasurer of the mosque committee:

'On this question of the responsibilities of fathers and mothers and according to the conditions of this area – truly, me myself, what I have seen with my own eyes is that compared to us men, women are those who do things. A man, if you need him, he is always out, whereas the woman is the one at home, taking care of the cooking and all other household affairs. If you talk about the progress of young people, however, the fault is on our side – we, the men. We are not firm and resolute. Children look to their mothers and they are closer to her but if things go wrong at home she will say, wait until your father returns. However, actually we are defeated, we can't deliver. We might have two or three growing children, but when we get up in the mornings we go about our business and don't concern ourselves with whether they eat or not – we don't even ask why they were not eating with us the night before. We come home, we eat, we sleep, and in the morning we have no 'programme' to assure ourselves that the children are cared for – we leave it all to mama. We give orders, we are 'dictators' in the home.

Fathers should eat with their children, make sure that they go to school, assess their development. At the end of the year, the child perhaps fails at school, and the father doesn't even know! You don't know he has failed maths, history, geography – you have no idea!

So this is why I support the view that women take the heavier burden, and do more of the work in the family, than we men. All the work, cultivating, looking after the cows, the hens – all this work she must do. After all the work at home she goes out to cut grass for the cows, and then she's off to the farm. And if-' (his next words are drowned out by clapping and ululations from the women and Jamal). 'And then let's say it reaches Saturday it should be my responsibility to buy the soap for washing the clothes. Am I there? Or am I out? And maybe at the end of the

week there are clothes to repair, the child's uniform is torn and so on –
but do we involve ourselves? We don't. Saturday we say 'it's the week-
end', and we come rolling home at ten or eleven at night. Do we ask for a
report on what is going on at home? No!... And what I know about this
village is that there are more bars in the area than cafes, and that there is
no government control of men's freedom or responsibilities. It is not
surprising that young men are found roaming about at night, spreading
AIDS or breaking into people's houses. Fathers don't even know their
own children and have to call them: 'You! what's-your-name!'.

Even Ali is conceding the tenor of this – older men can unite around
criticism of young men's behaviour, blaming them for AIDS, even if this
means accepting that some of it must be related to their upbringing.

In care and support, as well as prevention, it is therefore necessary to confront
prevailing gender relations and, so far as possible, draw connections between the
way gender ideologies are embedded within both the sphere of intimate relations
and the legislation, policy and practice of the wider society. How far collective
activity around AIDS can progress a broader change in gender relations is difficult to assess. But work in this area opens up and demands consideration of the
links between the interpersonal and the societal.

Can greater economic security empower more generally?

One important question here relates to women's economic position and the
importance of focusing on income generation as an appropriate intervention
for increasing women's protection against HIV. If economic dependence on
men, whether in marriage or within the market economy, is a factor underlying women's vulnerability, how far does greater economic autonomy serve
of itself to 'empower' women by reducing their level of subordination –
whether in the larger society or in interpersonal relations? At the sharp end,
greater economic security and increased economic autonomy will certainly
give women more choices so that they need not find themselves with only
their sex to sell in order to ensure sustenance of themselves and their children.
But does independent economic security of itself 'solve' the problem? How
far does it impact on other gendered power relations, and particularly those
which govern intimate relations?

Whether economically independent or not, both women and men desire
relations of intimacy. In the context of AIDS some may have second thoughts
about entering or staying in such relationships, with women having greater
cause for concern knowing that men are more likely to have multiple partners.
In one focus group discussion in Mansa, for example, a debate opened up
about whether having a husband was 'worth it', with one woman declaring 'If

I had what I wanted, if I had enough money to have what I wanted, I would not marry'. However, if not a husband, she conceded that: 'I might have a child',[19] leading back to the contradictions which AIDS throws up.

The problem for economically independent women remains how to protect themselves in relations of intimacy, not least, but not only, when trying to conceive. An insistence on the use of condoms by women can be sabotaged – or so it has been suggested by stories about men putting holes in condoms or cutting off their ends – as though to reaffirm who is really in charge (Hart *et al.*, 1999). However apocryphal such stories, they speak to the intransigence of gendered power relations. Reid's (n.d.) comment that, whatever women's class position, age, legal rights 'or any other socio-economic variable', 'they share a doubt that their words will influence the behaviour of their men or the dynamics of their relationships', makes much the same point. Economic autonomy implies greater choice; higher levels of education may afford women greater skills and the higher level of education of their partners may make them more amenable to reasoned discussion and verbal negotiation. However, there is no direct causal link back from higher class position, higher educational qualifications or greater economic autonomy to a transformation of gendered power relations in intimate social systems, or at least none that has been conclusively demonstrated to date. Nor should we forget that women's greater economic autonomy also allows for more sexual freedom (especially noted in Rungwe), which can fuel greater risk. In the end, women's enhanced bargaining power or reasoned arguments about mutual danger may cause gendered power relations to bend. But the question is still how to fully transform them.

Crossing lines of power

It is evident from the Lushoto case study that women have diverse interests. They may be as capable as men of hi-jacking an AIDS initiative, and preventing those among their number who are most vulnerable from gaining purchase on an empowering agenda. This case also illustrates the problems associated with attempts to build initiatives around and for those most vulnerable and least knowledgeable about the dangers of AIDS. The very lack of skills and the vulnerability of the female school leavers who were recruited to this project engendered a passivity; the prevailing lines of authority along lines of age as well as gender made them mute in the face of the older, dynamic woman who was the group's patron. They dared not cross these lines.

The experience of the Natweshe group in Mansa, where women invited men to join partly in order to enlist their support and their labour, but additionally in the hope that they would be recipients of AIDS messages, is also instructive. The Natweshe women found it difficult to achieve a level of equality within the club when this patently did not obtain outside of it.

Both of these examples underline the importance of ensuring that an initiative remains with those most at risk, those on the receiving end of the dominance/subordination continuum, so that the collective experience serves to give them new skills, knowledge and possibilities for protection. Yet this can entail its own difficulties. One is precisely the fact that those most vulnerable are also least visible, least in possession of the skills needed to progress an initiative, least confident and, often, least seen as deserving of attention or external resources. Given this situation, paternalistic models are all too often adopted, as in the case of the Lisach group in Mansa. While often couched in the spirit of benevolence and not without value, their impact may be limited unless methodologies enabling the 'target group' to become self-reliant are put in place.

As the Lushoto example also illustrates, prevailing relations of power can be reasserted when attempts are made to push forward those in positions of subordination. This points to a dilemma posed more generally by strategies of empowerment. Attempts to alter power relations are likely to be resisted by those in positions of dominance, if such attempts threaten their position of relative privilege and access to resources.

Bringing men in

What then of strategies which bring men in or involve men in addressing their own role in the progress of the epidemic? What organisational mechanisms or methodologies may be useful here? As noted in Chapter 1, emphasis has recently been placed on men's responsibility, and on culturally-condoned male sexual behaviours and sexual practices which may be harmful to women and, in the case of AIDS, manifestly deadly. To the extent that male behaviours not only put their partners in danger, but themselves as well, it is in men's interest to change that behaviour – as it is in women's interest to assist them in doing so. The question is how, in what way and at whose initiative.

To focus on men as key to halting the epidemic is not to deny that many men have taken on board messages about AIDS and that, even if women predominate at grass roots level, there are many highly committed men involved in AIDS work. What must also be emphasised is the extent to which change has begun to occur. Even if not as quickly as required, and even if our initial surveys revealed instances not just of denial but of a disturbing disregard of the level of danger which exists ('I may be tempted to have sex when I travel'; 'I don't always use a condom with my girl-friends'[20]), the threat represented by AIDS has induced change in attitudes and behaviour. Declarations by men that they had cut down on sexual part-ners, used protection, and 'respected themselves' were common. Large numbers of male respondents to demographic and health surveys similarly claim to have changed their behaviour in the face of AIDS, by reducing the number of sexual partners, sticking to one partner, using means of protection, or abstaining from sex (Central Statistical Office, Zambia, 1997).[21] Young people in particular appear increasingly willing to use condoms.[22] While such claims may be over-stated, behaviour – especially male behaviour – is increasingly held up to inspection.

As was indicated in the chapter on Kapulanga, blame is cast on all sides, its object varying according to the accuser's gender and age. In that case it was mainly women and 'rich' men who were regarded as most blameworthy; in Rungwe it was young people and particularly independent women. In a focus group discussion among traditional healers in Kanyama, however, several of the male participants acknowledged the way in which norms of masculinity must be held up to scrutiny: 'To make a very honest contribution', said one, 'we the men, are the problem'. Another concurred: 'I am a man, but I cannot shield myself from this blame. Talking about HIV/AIDS infection, the people who are primarily responsible are the men. It is not practicable for me to flirt around with other women hoping that I will use a condom with my wife …men are the ones who make propositions to women'.[23]

The question is, what can and what should men do? Is it enough to hope for individual realisation of the way in which masculine norms pose danger in the era of AIDS, or is collective action on the part of men – separately or jointly with women – in order? When asked what could be done about AIDS, one of the participants in a group of older men in Mansa said that women should form groups to teach each other about AIDS. When pressed, what could *they* do, the response of another was that he would change his behaviour by limiting the arena of his personal sexual activity, while leaving intact broad norms of masculine behaviour: 'men need to stop drinking from bars: It's better you send your child to buy beer and you drink it at home. When you feel like sleeping with a woman you can just call your wife'. His depiction of unquestioning submission by his wife was immediately challenged by other men in the group, however. 'But she will refuse', said one. 'How can she refuse?', asked the first man, 'she is my wife' 'Because you are smelling of beer', was the reply, drawing the sardonic laughter of the others.[24]

Another example of norms being questioned can be seen among some young people actively seeking to steep themselves in 'life skills' which might strengthen their resolve and increase their chances of survival in what can only be seen as a frightening environment. Sometimes underpinned by religious faith, these invariably stress positive peer support,[25] and emphasise a positive attitude and self control. Even if not explicitly formulated as such, these initiatives could be developed further to incorporate a reformulation of notions of masculinity, with self discipline and restraint seen as strengths and a need to demonstrate sexual conquest a weakness. Such a reformulation could potentially be framed either in terms of male responsibility or self-preservation, or indeed in terms of a mutuality of respect on the part of both males and females. The nuances of difference are crucial, however. Male responsibility may be a valued objective. Yet if configured as paternalism, it can reproduce relations of dominance and subordination. A strategy which stresses equality in aspirations for life, mutual respect between men and women, mutual responsibility and mutual benefit from intimate relations will have far more profound effect.

Women setting agendas

To this end, while collective action and collective learning, and indeed positive peer support, can usefully be fostered among men and within mixed groups, there is still place for women's groups to continue to define objectives and to ensure that a genuine mutuality of interests is kept to the fore. Women need to be vigilant to ensure that prevailing gender relations are not simply reproduced by new strategies which leave them having to depend on the heightened insight and assumed responsibility of individual men. Deeper structural changes are needed, especially a transformation of gender relations. The paradox offering promise is that, although the nature and severity of its impact is a consequence of inequalities of power, AIDS can serve as a leveller of conflicting interests. Both rich and poor are among those afflicted. If women are most vulnerable, men are not spared. AIDS threatens the future by claiming the lives of the young. In this sense the epidemic exerts a strong persuasive influence, illustrating the illusory nature of any vested interest in maintaining a status quo which can bring harm to so many.

Concluding comments: is there a model on offer?

Our study was partly directed toward trying to assess – through looking at several examples across two countries – whether a model involving the harnessing of women's organising capacities could be devised and which might have general application. This was always an ambitious aim and no single model has materialised. What 'works' depends on a wide range of variables, associated with the specific way men and women relate to each other in a given economic, cultural and political context, the nature of the social divisions within a given situation and the particular way that AIDS highlights and insinuates itself into a community in respect of them. However, we *have* identified a set of general principles which can inform the devising of strategies so as to ensure their greater effectiveness in meeting objectives and their congruence with broader changes in those 'deep structures', including gender relations, which drive the epidemic.

In AIDS work what is crucial, we argue, is not just that collective activity meets immediate objectives of extending awareness or giving support, but that it becomes an instrument of collective struggle against the factors which drive the epidemic. Initially, what is important is that it impact on participants, giving them not just additional skills and a greater sense of self worth, but also addressing the risks they face in their own lives and their own relationships. What is crucial, moreover, is that links be made and pursued between change at individual and societal levels, that short term protection is consistent with and promotes, rather than undermines, long term objectives and that the meeting of immediate practical interests is congruent with strategic goals.

Interventions need to expose and challenge those relations of power which drive the epidemic but must also stress the mutuality of interest in their transformation across lines of cleavage. They must therefore take account of social divisions within communities and power relations within personal relationships. They must begin with and ensure that the initiative remains with the 'disadvantaged' in order to challenge disabling divisions and 'harmful' power relations; but they must also seek means of building alliances and addressing the mutuality of interests transcending current divisions. They must take account of the way in which economic relations and cost/benefit calculations are necessarily embedded in AIDS work. While voluntarism is to be encouraged, it is important to reveal costs incurred and to counter the assumption that women's time and caring skills, in particular, are free goods or natural community resources. Moreover, particularly in the case of women, mechanisms of collective compensation should be sought which ensure individual survival and promote individual security.

For all its destructive power, the AIDS epidemic harbours strong liberatory potential, both in respect of transforming gender relations and in encouraging greater democratic participation. To be most effective, strategies for protection and prevention must promote greater inclusiveness and address those injustices, inequalities and human rights deficits which fuel the epidemic. We have emphasised the importance of structuring interventions so as to reveal what needs to be changed and to move in the direction of that required change. But many outstanding issues regarding the mechanics of practice remain. Organisational methodologies relating to women's collective action can be specified. But further consideration needs to be given to how to bring in men and how, organisationally or otherwise, to tackle forms of masculinity whose harm is made fatally manifest in the context of AIDS.

Notes

1 Lyons (1997) notes that promiscuity is a problematic term in AIDS discourse, having multiple meanings both within local African contexts and as applied by the (often external) scientific community. It is the discourse which is being described here, with recognition that, while specific meanings of the term vary, reference to promiscuity is invariably laden with moral connotations.

2 See for example Cornwall and Lindisfarne (1994) and discussion in Bujra (2000c). The vignette in Box 4 illustrates distinctive differences in masculine stance, even from men in the same village.

3 Lushoto, Maisha interviewee, 1999.

4 Kapulanga focus group, women aged 15–20, 30 April 1996, facilitator, A. Sikwibele.

5 Mansa focus group, women aged 30–54, 9 April 1996, facilitator, T. Chabala.

6 Correspondence, A. Kunda, 12 November 1996.

7 Kanyama focus group, women aged 15–19, April 1996, facilitator A. Mkandawire.

8 Ibid..

9 Mansa focus group, older men, May 1996, facilitator, T. Chabala.

10   Kanyama focus group, women aged 21–45, PUSH Project Workers, 24 June 1996; facilitator A. Mkandawire.
11   Mansa focus group, women aged 30–54, 9 April 1996, facilitator, T. Chabala.
12   Kanyama focus group, traditional healers, 25 April 1996, facilitator A. Mkandawire. US dollar equivalents are based on the exchange rate at the time the focus group was held.
13   Mansa focus group, older women, 23 May 1996, facilitator, T. Chabala.
14   Many examples can be given, as recorded in annual reports of the Muchinka Teen Centre, evaluation of peer education projects and anti-AIDS clubs or reviews of CHEP's activities (Mouli, 1991; Hughes-d'Aeth, 1998).
15   Mbilinyi and Mwabuki (1996) refer in similar context to personal and organisational needs.
16   See, for example, statements and press releases accompanying the UN Security Council's discussion of AIDS in Africa on 10 January 2000 (UNAIDS, 2000a), building in turn on a range of other documents and initiatives such as the Africa Partnership against HIV/AIDS and the World Bank's (1999) undertaking to intensify action against AIDS in Africa.
17   Address by J. Wolfensohn, President of the World Bank, to the UN Security Council, 10 January 2000, http://www.unaids.org, press release.
18   Interview, Mansa, 8 August 1999.
19   Mansa, group discussion, 12 April 1996.
20   Kanyama survey respondents.
21   See also UNAIDS/WHO (2000a,b) for data on changes in reported use of condoms by age and sex in Tanzania and Zambia. Both countries also report a fall in the proportion of sexually active people claiming to have had more than one sexual partner over the previous 12 months (ibid.).
22   Our baseline surveys showed a relationship between age and willingness to use condoms across all three sites in Zambia and the combined Tanzanian sample.
23   Kanyama focus group, traditional healers, 25 April 1996, facilitator, A. Mkandawire.
24   Mansa focus group, men aged 46 and over, 23 May 1996, facilitator, T. Chabala.
25   Examples include the Youth Alive movement in Zambia and elsewhere (Siame, 1998) and a programme of action developed by the Lusaka Interfaith HIV/AIDS Networking Group (Banda *et al.*, n.d.). Some of these same features are also incorporated in the Stepping Stones programme developed by ActionAID and the work of Fr Joinet in Tanzania (1994a,b).

Bibliography

af-aids:hivnet, 22 September 1999. young men also at risk.

af-aids:hivnet.ch [411] (22 September 1999), ICASA Track Three – HIV/AIDS Spread 2 [362].

Agenda (1998) Special issue: *AIDS, Counting the Cost*, 39.

Aggleton, P. and Warwick, I. (1999) 'Community responses to AIDS', Part 2, Sex and youth: contextual factors affecting risk for HIV/AIDS, a comparative analysis of multi-site studies in developing countries, Geneva: UNAIDS. Online. Available HTTP: http://www.unaids.org.

AIDS Analysis Africa, 7 February 1997.

Akeroyd, A. (1997) 'Sociocultural aspects of AIDS in Africa: occupational and gender issues', in G. Bond, J. Kreniske, I. Susser and J. Vincent (eds), *AIDS in Africa and the Caribbean*, Boulder, Colorado: Westview Press.

Ahlemeyer, H. and Ludwig, D. (1997) 'Norms of communication and communication as a norm in the intimate social system', in L. Van Campenhoudt, M. Cohen, G. Guizzardi and D. Hausser (eds), *Sexual Interactions and HIV Risk, new conceptual perspectives in European Research*, London: Taylor & Francis.

Alcorn, K. (1988) 'Illness, metaphor and AIDS', in P. Aggleton and H. Homans (eds), *Social Aspects of AIDS*, Barcombe: Falmer Press.

Ankrah, E. M. (1991) 'AIDS and the social side of health', *Social Science and Medicine* 32, 9: 967–980.

Ankrah E. M. (1996) 'AIDS, socio-economic decline and health: a double crisis for the African woman', in L. Sherr, C. Hankins and L. Bennett (eds), *AIDS as a Gender Issue, Psychological Perspectives*, London: Taylor & Francis.

Ankrah, E. M., Schwartz, M. and Miller, J. (1996) 'Care and support systems', in L. Long and E. M. Ankrah (eds), *Women's experience with HIV/AIDS, an international perspective*, New York: Columbia University Press.

Baden, S. and Wach, H. (1998) 'Gender, HIV/AIDS transmission and impacts: a review of issues and evidence', Bridge, Report No. 47, Institute of Development Studies, University of Sussex. Online. Available HTTP: http://www.ids.ac.uk/bridge.

Baggaley, R., Sulwe, J., Kelly, M., Ndovi Macmillan, M. and Godfrey-Faussett, P. (1996) 'HIV counsellors' knowledge, attitudes and vulnerabilities to HIV in Lusaka, Zambia, 1994', *AIDS Care* 8, 2: 155–166.

Ballard, R. (1999) 'Challenges for HIV/STD research in Africa', Paper for plenary session presented at the XI International Conference on AIDS and STDs in Africa, Lusaka, 12–16 September.

Banda, M., Canteen, A., Fube, F., Hachonda, H., Hobbs, A., Iman, I., Kasanga, L., *et al.* (n.d.) *Treasuring the Gift, how to handle God's gift of sex, sexual health learning activities for religious youth groups*, compiled by Lusaka Interfaith HIV/AIDS Networking Group Lusaka, Project Concern International (Zambia).

Barnett, T. and Blaikie, P. (1992) *AIDS in Africa, Its Present and Future Impact*, London: Belhaven Press.

Barongo, L., Rugemalila, J., Gabone, R. and Senkoro, K. (1992) 'The epidemiology of HIV infection in adolescents in Kagera region', Poster presented at International Conference on AIDS, Amsterdam, July 1992.

Bassett, M. and Mhloyi, M. (1991) 'Women and AIDS in Zimbabwe, the making of the epidemic', *International Journal of Health Services* 21, 1: 143–156.

Bayley, A. (1984) 'Aggressive Kaposi's sarcoma in Zambia, 1983', *The Lancet* 1, 2: 1318–1320.

Baylies, C. (1999a) 'Community based research on AIDS in the context of global inequalities', Paper presented to a Symposium on HIV/AIDS in Africa: reviewing the past, understanding the present and charting the future, Urbana, Illinois, 14–17 July.

Baylies, C. (1999b) 'International partnership in the fight against AIDS, addressing need and redressing injustice?' *Review of African Political Economy* 26, 81: 387–394.

Baylies, C. and Bujra, J. (1995) 'Discourses of power and empowerment in the fight against HIV/AIDS in Africa', in P. Aggleton, P. Davies and G. Hart (eds), *AIDS, Safety, Sexuality and Risk*, London: Taylor and Francis.

Baylies, C., Bujra, J., *et al.* (1999) 'Rebels at risk, young women and the shadow of AIDS' in C. Becker, J.-P. Dozon, C. Obbo and M. Toure (eds), *Experiencing and Understanding AIDS in Africa*, Dakar/Paris: Codesria/Editions Karthala/IRD.

Becker, C., Dozon, J.-P., Obbo, C. and Toure, M. (eds) (1999) *Experiencing and Understanding AIDS in Africa*, Dakar/Paris: Codesria/ Editions Karthala/IRD.

Berer, M. (1999) 'HIV/AIDS, pregnancy and maternal mortality: implications for care', in M. Berer and T. K. Sundari Ravindran (eds), *Safe Motherhood Initiatives: Critical Issues*, London: Blackwell Science for Reproductive Health Matters.

Berer, M. and Ray, S. (eds) (1993) *Women and HIV/AIDS: an international resource book*, London: AHRTAG/Pandora Press.

Blinkhoff, P., Bukanga, E., Syamalevwe X. and Williams, G. (1999) *Under the Mupundu Tree, Volunteers in Home Care for People with HIV/AIDS and TB in Zambia's Copperbelt* Strategies for Hope Series, No. 14, London: ActionAid.

Bond, G. and Vincent, J. (1997) 'Community based organizations in Uganda: a youth initiative', in G. Bond, J. Kreniske, I. Susser and J. Vincent (eds), *AIDS in Africa and the Caribbean*, Boulder, Colorado: Westview Press, (1997).

Bond, G., Kreniske, J., Susser, I. and Vincent, J. (eds) (1997) *AIDS in Africa and the Caribbean*, Boulder, Colorado: Westview Press.

Bond, V. (1997) '"Between a rock and a hard place": applied anthropology and AIDS research on a commercial farm in Zambia', *Health Transition Review* 7 suppl: 69–83.

Boulton, M. (ed) (1994) *Challenge and Innovation, Methodological Advances in Social Research on HIV/AIDS*, London: Taylor & Francis.

British Tanzania Newsletter, May 1999.

Bujra, J. (2000a) 'Risk and trust: unsafe sex, gender and AIDS in Tanzania', in P. Caplan (ed), *Risk Revisited*, London: Pluto Press.

Bujra, J. (2000b) *Serving Class, Masculinity and the Feminisation of Domestic Service in Tanzania*, London: International African Institute.

Bujra, J. (2000c) 'Targeting men for a change: AIDS discourse and action in Africa', *Agenda* 44 (Durban).

Bujra, J. and Baylies, C. (1999) 'Solidarity and stress: gender and local mobilization in Tanzania and Zambia', in P. Aggleton, G. Hart and P. Davies (eds), *Families and Communities Responding to AIDS*, London: UCL Press.

Burkey, S. (1993) *People First, A Guide to Self-Reliant Participatory Rural Development*, London: Zed Books.

Bury, J. (1991) 'Women and the AIDS epidemic, some medical facts and figures', in J. Bury, V. Morrison and S. McLachlan (eds), *Working with Women and AIDS*, London: Routledge, Tavistock.

Campbell, C. and Williams, B. (1999) 'Beyond the biomedical and behavioural: towards an integrated approach to HIV prevention in the Southern African mining industry', *Social Science and Medicine* 48: 1625–1639.

Campbell, I. (1989) 'Impact of AIDS and a community based response at Chikankata Hospital, a two year review', Paper presented at the Integrated AIDS Management Conference, Nairobi, 21–24 May.

Campbell, I. and Williams, G. (1990) *AIDS Management: an integrated approach*, London: ActionAid, in association with AMREF and World in Need.

Campbell, T. and Kelly, M. (1995) 'Women and AIDS in Zambia: a review of the psychosocial factors implicated in the transmission of HIV', *AIDS Care* 7, 3: 365–373.

Caplan, G. (1970) *The Elites of Barotseland 1878–1969: a Political History of Zambia's Western Province*, London: C. Hurst.

Caplan, P. (1978) 'Women's organisations in Madras city, India', in P. Caplan and J. Bujra (eds), *Women United, Women Divided*, London: Tavistock.

Carael, M. (1995) 'Sexual behaviour', in J. Cleland and B. Ferry (eds), *Sexual Behaviour and AIDS in the Developing World*, London: Taylor and Francis.

Carovano, K. (1991) 'More than mothers and whores: redefining the AIDS prevention needs of women', *International Journal of Health Services* 21, 1: 131–142.

Carovano, K. (1995) HIV and the challenges facing men', Issues Paper #15, UNDP, HIV and Development Programme. Online. Available HTTP: http://www.undp.issues.

Carpenter, L., Kamali, A., Ruberantwari, A., Malamba, S. and Whitworth, A. (1999) 'Rates of HIV-1 transmission within marriage in rural Uganda in relation to the HIV sero-status of the partners', *AIDS* 13: 1083–1089.

Carpenter, L., Nakiyingi, J., Ruberantwari, A., Malamba, S., Kamali, A. and Whitworth, J. (1997) 'Estimates of the impact of HIV infection on fertility in a rural Ugandan population cohort', *Health Transition Review* 7 suppl 2: 113–126.

Central Statistical Office [Zambia] and Ministry of Health and Macro International Inc. (1997) *Zambia Demographic and Health Survey 1996* Calverton, Maryland: Central Statistical Office and Macro International, Inc.

Chabal, P. and Daloz, J.-P. (1999) *Africa Works: Disorder as Political Instrument*, London: The International African Institute.

Chalowandya, C. M. and Chitomfwa, P. B. (1995a) 'Anti AIDS club monitoring and evaluation report for Central Province' unpublished report.

Chalowandya, C. M. and Chitomfwa, P. B. (1995b) 'Eastern Province monitoring and evaluation report of Anti AIDS clubs, case study of Petauke and Nyimba', unpublished report.

Chela, C., Campbell, I. and Siankanga, Z. (1989) 'Clinical care as part of integrated AIDS management in a Zambian rural community', *AIDS Care* 1, 3: 319–325.

Christian Council of Tanzania (CCT) (1987) Kimbunga Baseline Printers.

Cleland, J., Ali, M. and Capo-Chichi, V. (1998) 'Post-partum sexual abstinence in West Africa: implications for AIDS-control and family planning programmes', *AIDS* 13: 125–131.

Cleland J. and Ferry, B. (1995) *Sexual Behaviour and AIDS in the Developing World*, London: Taylor and Francis.

Cohen, D. (1998a) 'The HIV epidemic and sustainable human development', Issues Paper # 29, UNDP, HIV and Development Programme. Online. Available HTTP: http://www.undp.org. hiv.

Cohen, D. (1998b) 'Poverty and HIV/AIDS in Sub-Saharan Africa', Issues Paper, # 27, UNDP, HIV and Development Programme. Online. Available HTTP: http://www.undp.org. hiv.

Cohen, D. (1998c) 'Socio-economic causes and consequences of the HIV epidemic in southern Africa: a case study of Namibia', Issues Paper # 31, UNDP, HIV and Development Programme. Online. Available HTTP: http://www.undp.org. hiv.

Cohen, D. and Reid, E. (1996) 'The vulnerability of women: is this a useful construct for policy and programming', Issues Paper #28, UNDP, HIV and Development Programme. Online. Available HTTP: http://www.undp.org.hiv.

Commins, S. (1999) 'NGOs: Ladles in the global soup kitchen?' *Development in Practice* 9, 5: 619–622.

Cornwall, A. and Lindisfarne, N. (1994) *Dislocating Masculinity: Comparative Ethnographies*, London: Routledge.

Daily News (Tanzania), 6 June 1996.

Davies, D. H. (ed) (1971) *Zambia in Maps*, London: University of London Press.

de Bruyn, M. (1992) 'Women and AIDS in developing countries', *Social Science and Medicine* 34, 3: 249–262.

Des Jarlais, D. and Caraël, M. (1999) 'Behavioral and social science', Overview, *AIDS* 13 suppl A: S235-S237.

Deverell, K. (1997) 'Professional and sexual identity in gay and bisexual men's HIV prevention', in P. Aggleton, P. Davies and G. Hart (eds), *AIDS: Activism and Alliances*, London: Taylor & Francis.

Doyal, L. (1994) 'HIV and AIDS: putting women on the global agenda', in L. Doyal, J. Naidoo and T. Wilton (eds), *AIDS, Setting a Feminist Agenda*, London: Taylor and Francis.

Dozon, P. and Chabal, J.-P. (1999) *Africa Works: Disorder as Political Instrument*, London: International African Institute.

du Guerny, J. and Sjöberg, E. (1993) 'Inter-relationship between gender relations and the HIV/AIDS epidemic: some possible considerations for policies and programmes', *AIDS* 7: 1027–1034.

du Lou, A., Msellati, P., Yao, A., Noba, V., Viho, I., Ramon, R., Welffens-Ekra, C. and Dabis, F. (1999) 'Impaired fertility in HIV-1-infected pregnant women: a clinic-based survey in Abidjan, Cote d'Ivoire, 1997', *AIDS* 13: 517–521.

Edwards, M. and Hulme, D. (1995) 'NGO performance and accountability in the post-Cold War world', *Journal of International Development* 7, 6: 849–856.

Elson, D. (1995) 'Male bias in the development process: an overview', in D. Elson (ed), *Male Bias in the Development Process*, (2nd edn), Manchester: Manchester University Press.

Essex, M. (1999) 'Vaccine initiatives in and for Africa', Paper for plenary session presented at the XI International Conference on AIDS and STDs in Africa, Lusaka, 12–16 September.

Farmer, P. (1999) 'AIDS and social scientists: critical reflections', in C. Becker, J.-P. Dozon, C. Obbo and M. Toure (eds), *Experiencing and Understanding AIDS in Africa*, Dakar/Paris: Codesria/ Editions Karthala/IRD.

Foreman, M. (ed) (1999) *AIDS and Men, taking risks or taking responsibility?* London: Panos/Zed.

Foreman, M. (1999) 'Men, sex and HIV', in M. Foreman (ed), *AIDS and Men, taking risks or taking responsibility?* London: Panos/Zed.

Foster, S. (n.d.) 'Cost and burden of AIDS on the Zambian health care system: policies to mitigate the impact on health services', Paper prepared for USAID.

Foster, S., Chibomba, F., Mukonka, V. and O'Connell, A. (1991) 'Costs of AIDS counselling and home based care at Monze District Hospital, Monze, Zambia', Paper presented at the WHO Workshop on Home and Community Based Care, Entebbe, Uganda, October.

Fuglesang, M. (1997) 'Lessons for life – past and present modes of sexuality education in Tanzanian society', *Social Science and Medicine* 44, 8: 1245–1254.

Fylkesnes, K. (1995) 'Overview of the HIV/AIDS situation in Zambia: patterns and trends', Paper presented at the 5th National AIDS Conference, Lusaka, May 1995.

Fylkesnes, K., Brunborg, H. and Msiska, R. (1994) *Zambia: the Current HIV/AIDS Situation – and Future Demographic Impact*, Background Paper 1, The Socio-economic Impact of AIDS, Lusaka: Ministry of Health.

Fylkesnes, K., Mubanga Musonda, R., Kasumba, K., Ndhlovu, Z., Mluanda, F., Kaetano, L. and Chipaila, C. (1997) 'The HIV epidemic in Zambia: socio-demographic prevalence patterns and indications of trends among childbearing women', *AIDS* 11: 339–345.

Fylkesnes, K., Musonda, R. M., Sichone, M., Ndhlovu, Z., Tembo, F., Monze, M., Kaetano, L., *et al.* (1999) abstract, 'Favourable changes in the HIV epidemic in Zambia in the 1990s', (late breaker abstract, XI Icasa) Online posting. Available e-mail: af-aids@hiv.ch, 437, 1 October 1999.

gender-aids@hivnet.ch, 15 October 1999.

gender-aids@hivnet.ch [574] (15 October 1999), Anti-AIDS Insurance for Rape Victims.

Gertzel, C. (1984) 'Western Province: tradition, economic deprivation and political alienation', in C. Gertzel, C. Baylies and M. Szeftel (eds), *The Dynamics of the One-Party State in Zambia*, Manchester: Manchester University Press.

Gibb, D. and Tess, B. (1999) 'Interventions to reduce mother-to-child transmission of HIV infection: new developments and current controversies', *AIDS* 13 suppl A: S93-S102.

Gluckman, M. (1941) *Economy of the Central Barotse Plain*, The Rhodes-Livingstone Papers, 7, The Rhodes-Livingstone Institute, Manchester: Manchester University Press.

Gluckman, M. (1951) 'The Lozi of Barotseland in North-western Rhodesia', in E. Colson and M. Gluckman (eds), *Seven Tribes of British Central Africa*, London: Oxford University Press.

Gluckman, M. (1955) *The Judicial Process among the Barotse of Northern Rhodesia*, Manchester: Manchester University Press.

Goetz, A. M. (1997) 'Local heroes: patterns of fieldworker discretion in implementing GAD policy in Bangladesh' in A. M. Goetz (ed), *Getting Institutions Right for Women in Development*, London: Zed Books.

Gordon, P. and Crehan K. (1999) 'Dying of sadness: gender, sexual violence and the HIV epidemic', Gender and the HIV Epidemic. New York: UNDP HIV and Development Programme. Online. Available HTTP: http://www.undp.org. hiv/genderlist.htm.

Gottemoeller, M. (1999) 'Microbicides: new hope for HIV protection', Paper presented at the XII International Conference on AIDS and STDs in Africa, Lusaka 12–16 September.

Government of Tanzania (1988) *Tanzania Census 1988*, Dar es Salaam: Bureau of Statistics.

Gregson, S., Zaba, B. and Garnett, G. (1999) 'Low fertility in women with HIV and the impact of the epidemic on orphanhood and early childhood mortality in sub-Saharan Africa', *AIDS* 13 suppl A: S249-S257.

Gregson, S., Zhuwau, T., Anderson, R. and Changiwana, S. (1998) 'Is there evidence for behaviour change in response to AIDS in rural Zimbabwe', *Social Science and Medicine* 46, 1: 321–333.

Guardian, 4 January 1999.

Hall, R. (1965) *Zambia*, London: Pall Mall Press.

Hamlin, J. and Reid, E. (1991) 'Women, the HIV epidemic and human rights: a tragic imperative', HIV and Development Programme, Issues Paper #8, UNDP. Online. Available: HTTP: (http://www.undp.org/hiv/issues.htm.

Harrison, E. (1997) 'Fish, feminists and the FOA: translating ''gender'' through different institutions in the development process' in A. M. Goetz (ed), *Getting Institutions Right for Women in Development*, London: Zed Books.

Hart, G., Pool, R., Green, G., Harrison, S., Nyanzi, S. and Whitworth, J. (1999) 'Women's attitudes to condoms and female-controlled means of protection against HIV and STDs in South-Western Uganda', *AIDS Care* 11, 6: 687–698.

Hartwig (1991) 'The politics of AIDS in Tanzania: gender perceptions and the challenges for educational strategies', unpublished MA Thesis, Clark University, Massachusetts.

Heise, L. and Elias, C. (1995) 'Transforming AIDS prevention to meet women's needs: a focus on developing countries', *Social Science and Medicine* 40, 7: 931–943.

Hira, S., Mangrola, G., Mwale, C., Chintu, C., *et al*. (1990) 'Apparent vertical transmission of human immunodeficiency virus type 1 by breastfeeding in Zambia', *Journal of Paediatrics* 117 (3): 421–424.

Hoelscher, M., Riedner, G., Hemed, Y., Wagner, H., Korte, R. and von Sonnenburg, F. (1994) 'Estimating the number of HIV transmissions through reused syringes and needles in the Mbeya Region, Tanzania', *AIDS* 8: 1609–1615.

Holland, J., Ramazanoglu, C., Sharpe, S. and Thompson, R. (1992) 'Pressure, resistance, empowerment: young women and the negotiation of safer sex', in P. Aggleton, P. Davies and G. Hart (eds), *AIDS, rights, risks and reason*, London: Falmer Press.

Holland, J., Ramazanoglu, C., Sharpe, S. and Thompson, R. (1998) *The Male in the Head, Young People, Heterosexuality and Power*, London: Tufnell Press.

Hughes-d'Aeth, A. (1998) Evaluation of peer education projects, report produced for Unicef, Zambia YE-502-03, Learning Education Project.

Ishumi, A. (1984) *The Urban Jobless in Eastern Africa*, Uppsala: Scandinavian Institute of African Studies.

Jackson, C. (1997) 'Actor orientation and gender relations a participatory project interface' in A. M. Goetz (ed), *Getting Institutions Right for Women in Development*, London: Zed Books.

Jewkes, R. (1999), 'Forcing the issue: relationship dynamics and adolescent fertility in South Africa', Paper presented at the Fertility in Southern Africa Workshop, London, 22–24 September.

Joinet, B. (1994a) *The Challenge of AIDS in East Africa, Part One: Basic Facts*, Dar es Salaam.

Joinet, B. (1994b) *The Challenge of AIDS in East Africa Part Two: Prevention and Survivors*, Dar es Salaam.

Kabeer, N. (1994) *Reversed Realities, Gender Hierarchies in Development Thought*, London: Verso.

Kaihula, N. (1995) *The Effects of Wives' Economic Power on Gender Relationships in Tanzania Households*, unpublished MA thesis, Department of Development Studies, University of Dar es Salaam.

Kaihula, N. (1996) 'Religion and HIV/AIDS; issues on community and church responses over protective strategies', Paper presented at the Gender and HIV/AIDS Workshop, Dar es Salaam, 22–23 August.

Kaijage, T. (1991) WAMATA: self-help at the Tanzanian grassroots', *AIDS Analysis Africa* 1, 4: 12.

Kaijage, T. (1993) 'WAMATA: People striving to control the spread of AIDS, Tanzania', in M. Berer with S. Ray (eds), *Women and HIV/AIDS: an international resource book*, London: AHRTAG/Pandora Press.

Kaijage, T. (1995) 'There are lessons to be learned', in E. Reid (ed), *HIV and AIDS: The Global Interconnection*, West Hertford, Connecticutt: Kumarian Press.

Kaleeba, N. (1991) *We Miss You All: AIDS in the Family*, Women and AIDS Support Network, Harare.

Kaler, A. (1999) '''It's some kind of empowerment'': the ambiguity of the female condom as a marker of female empowerment', Paper presented at the Fertility in Southern Africa Workshop, London, 22–24 September.

Kalindile, R. and Mbilinyi, M. (1991) 'Grassroot struggles for women's advancement: the story of Rebeka Kalindile', in B. Koda and M. Ngaiza (eds), *The Unsung Heroines*, Dar es Salaam: Dar es Salaam University Press for WRDP.

Kalipenta, J. and Chalowandya, C. (1995) 'Southern Province peer education programme, groundwork report, pilot study areas: Mazabuka and Monze' (mimeo).

Kapiga, S. (1996) 'Determinants of multiple sexual partners and condom use among sexually active Tanzanians', *East African Medical Journal* 73, 7: 435–442.

Kapiga, S., Lyamuya, F., Lwihula, G. and Hunter, D. (1998) 'The incidence of HIV infection among women using family planning methods in Dar es Salaam, Tanzania', *AIDS* 12: 75–84.

Kapiga, S., Nachtigal, G. and Hunter, D. (1991) 'Knowledge of AIDS among secondary school pupils in Bagamoyo and Dar es Salaam, Tanzania', *AIDS* 5: 325–328.

Karl, M. (1995) *Women and Empowerment: Participation and Decision Making*, London: Zed Books.

Katapa, R. (1998) 'Nyakyusa teenage sexuality', in M. Rwebangira and R. Liljestrom (eds), *Haraka Haraka: Look Before You Leap*, Uppsala: Nordic African Institute.

Kiondo, A. (1993) 'Structural adjustment and non-governmental organisations in Tanzania: a case study', in P. Gibbon (ed), *Social Change and Economic Reform in Africa*, Uppsala: Nordiska Afrikainstitutet.

Kiwara, A. (1994) 'Structural adjustment programmes and health: gender implications', unpublished paper, Tanzania Gender Networking Programme (TGNP).

Klepp, K., Ndeki, S., Thuen, F., Leshabari, M. and Seha, A. (1994) 'AIDS education for primary school children in Tanzania, an evaluation study', *AIDS* 8: 1157–1162.

Koekkoek, M. and Steenbeck, E. (1995) 'Coordination constraints in Tanzania', *SafAIDS Bulletin*, 1: 15–16.

Kreniske, J. (1997) 'AIDS in the Dominican Republic, anthropological reflections on the social nature of disease', in G. Bond, J. Kreniske, I. Susser and J. Vincent (eds), (1997) *AIDS in Africa and the Caribbean*, Boulder, Colorado: Westview Press.

Kristeva, J. (1982) *The Dilemma of Horror*, New York: Columbia University Press.

Leroy, V., Van de Perre, P., Lepage, P., Saba, J., Nsengumuremyi, F., Simonon, A., Karita, E., Msellatti, P., Salamon, R. and Dabis, F. (1994) 'Seroincidence of HIV-1 infection in African women of reproductive age: a prospective cohort study in Kigali, Rwanda, 1988–1992', *AIDS* 8: 983–986.

Leshabari, M. and Kaaya, S. (1997) 'Bridging the information gap: sexual maturity and reproductive health problems among youth in Tanzania', *Health Transition Review* 7 suppl 3: 29–44.

Lewanika Hospital (1994) Records and statistics, Mongu.

Lie, G. T. and Biswalo, P. M. (1994) 'Perceptions of the appropriate HIV/AIDS counselling in Arusha and Kilimanjaro region of Tanzania: implications for hospital counselling', *AIDS Care* 6, 2: 139–151.

Liljestrom, R., Masanja, P., Rwebangira, M. and Urassa, E. (1998) 'Cultural conflicts and ambiguities', in M. Rwebangira and R. Liljestrom (eds), *Haraka Haraka... Look Before You Leap*, Uppsala: Nordic African Institute.

Lindenbaum, S. (1992) 'Knowledge and action in the shadow of AIDS', in G. Herdt and S. Lindenbaum (eds), *The Time of AIDS*, London: Sage.

Long, L. (1996) 'Introduction: counting women's experiences', in L. Long and M. Ankrah (eds), *Women's Experiences with HIV/AIDS, an International Perspective*, New York: Columbia University Press.

Lugalla, J. (1995) 'Structural adjustment policies and health policy in Tanzania, their impact on women's and children's health', *Review of African Political Economy* 63: 43–53.

Lyons, M. (1997) 'The point of view: perspectives on AIDS in Uganda', in G. Bond, J. Kreniske, I. Susser and J. Vincent (eds), *AIDS in Africa and the Caribbean*, Boulder, Colorado: Westview Press.

Maarugu, E. (Mansa District Health Services) (1995) January to December 1995 Annual Report, UNV Technical Support to Strengthen Community Oriented HIV/AIDS Care and Support Programmes, Mansa.

McNamara, R. (1991) 'Female genital, health and the risk of HIV transmission', Issues Paper No. 3, UNDP, HIV and Development Programme.

Macwan'gi, M., Sichone, M. and Kamanga, P. (1994) *Women and AIDS in Zambia, situation analysis and options for HIV/AIDS survival assistance*, Study commissioned by National AIDS Prevention and Control Programme and funded by SIDA, Lusaka.

Madavo, C. (1999) 'A new compact on AIDS', Address to the International Conference on AIDS and STDs in Africa, Lusaka, 12 September 1999.

Madrigal, J., Schifter, J. and Feldblum, P. J. (1998) 'Female condom acceptability among sex workers in Costa Rica', *AIDS Education & Prevention* 10, 2:105–113.

Madunagu, B. (1998) 'Curbing the spread of HIV/AIDS in Africa: a focus on women', in A. Gomez and D. Meacham (eds), *Women, Vulnerability and HIV/AIDS: A Human Rights Perspective*, Women's Health Collective/3.

Mainga, M. (1973) *Bulozi under the Luyana Kings: Political Evolution and State Formation in Pre-colonial Zambia*, London: Longmans.

Mann, J., Tarantola, D. and Netter, T. (eds) (1992) *AIDS in the World: A Global Report*, Cambridge, Massachusetts: Harvard University Press.

Mann, J. and Tarantola, D. (eds) (1996) *AIDS and the World II, Global Dimensions, Social Roots and Responses*, Oxford: Oxford University Press.

Mansa Hospital (1995) Records and statistics, Mansa.

Mascarenhas, O. and Mbilinyi, M. (1983) *Women in Tanzania: An Analytical Bibliography*, Uppsala: Scandinavian Institute of African Studies.

Mbilinyi, M. (1979) 'Contradictions in Tanzanian education reform', in A. Coulson (ed), *African Socialism in Practice: The Tanzanian Experience*, Nottingham: Spokesman.

Mbilinyi, M. (1989) '"This is an unforgettable business!" colonial state intervention in urban Tanzania', in J. Parpart and K. Staudt (eds), *Women and the State in Africa* Boulder, Colorado: Lynne Rienner.

Mbilinyi, M. (1991) *Big Slavery: Agribusiness and the Crisis in Women's Employment in Tanzania*, Dar es Salaam: Dar es Salaam University Press.

Mbilinyi, M. (1994) 'Gender and structural adjustment', paper presented to TGNP Symposium on Gender and Structural Adjustment, Dar es Salaam, 26 February 1994.

Mbilinyi, M. (1997) 'Impact of structural adjustment on women's employment in rural areas', unpublished report submitted to ILO Geneva.

Mbilinyi, M. and Mwabuki, J. (1996) 'NGOs and the struggle against HIV/AIDS', Paper presented to the Annual Gender Studies Conference, Dar es Salaam, 5–8 December.

Mbilinyi-Segule, N. (1999) 'The economic impact of HIV/AIDS on Tanzania's development', Dar es Salaam' unpublished report for the World Bank.

Melbye, M., Bayley, A. C., Manuwele, J. K., Clayden, S. A. and Blattner, R., Tedder, R., Njelesani, E., Mukelabai, K., Bowa, F., Levin, A., Weiss, R. and Bigger, R. (1986) 'Evidence for the heterosexual transmission and clinical manifestations of human immuno-deficiency virus infection and related conditions in Lusaka, Zambia', *The Lancet* 2: 1113–1115.

Mercer, C. (1999) 'Reconceptualising state-society relations in Tanzania: are NGOs "making a difference"?', *Area* 31, 3: 247–258.

Mgalla, Z. and Pool, R. (1997) 'Sexual relationships, condom use and risk perception among female bar workers in north-west Tanzania', *AIDS Care* 8, 4: 407–416.

Mgalla, Z., Schapink, D. and Ties Boerma, J. (1998) 'Protecting schoolgirls against sexual exploitation, a guardian programme in Mwanza, Tanzania', *Reproductive Health Matters* 6, 2: 19–30.

Ministry of Health, (Zambia) (1993) *Mobilization of Zambian Women in the Prevention and Control of AIDS*, Second Medium Term Plan, 1994–1998, Zambia National AIDS/STD/TB & Leprosy Programme, Lusaka.

Ministry of Health, (Zambia) (1997) *HIV/AIDS in Zambia, background, projections, impacts and interventions*, Lusaka.

Ministry of Health, (Zambia) NASTLP (1997) Assorted tables, Lusaka.

Mnyika, K., Klepp, K.I., Kvale, G., Schreiner, A. and Seha, A.M. (1995a) 'Condom awareness and use in the Arusha and Kilimanjaro regions, Tanzania: a population-based study', *AIDS Education and Prevention* 7, 5: 403–414.

Mnyika, K.S., Kvale, G. and Klepp, K.I. (1995b) 'Perceived function and barriers to condom use in Arusha and Kilimanjaro regions of Tanzania', *AIDS Care* 7, 5: 295–305.

Molyneux, M. (1985) 'Mobilisation without emancipation? Women's interests, the state and revolution in Nicaragua', *Feminist Studies* 11: 227–254.

Molyneux, M. (1998) 'Analysing women's movements', *Development and Change* 29: 219–245.

Moser, C. (1993) *Gender Planning and Development, theory, practice and training*, London: Routledge.

Mouli, V. C. (1991) 'A report of three and a half years of AIDS "health promotion" work on the Copperbelt Province, Zambia', unpublished report.

Mouli, V. C. (1992) *All Against AIDS, the Copperbelt Health Education Project, Zambia, strategies for hope*, No. 7, Oxford: ActionAid in association with AMREF and Christian Aid.

Msaky, I. and Kisesa, A. (1997) Report of inventory of the local institutions/NGOs and human resources for HIV/AIDS/STD Programmes in Tanzania, unpublished paper, Muhimbili Medical Centre, Dar es Salaam.

Msamanga (1999) Online posting. Available e-mail: af-aids@hivnet.ch (25 January 1995).

Mudenda, S. (ed) (1991) *Sharing the Challenge*, Report of the Second Zambian AIDS NGO Conference, Lusaka.

Mukonde, C. (1992) *Too Young to Die*, Lusaka: Zambia Educational Publishing House.

Mulenga, C. (1993) *Orphans, Widows and Widowers in Zambia: a situation analyhsis and options for HIV/AIDS survival assistance*, unpublished paper, Lusaka.

Mushinge, I. and Simwanza, T. (1996) 'The role of *Bana Cimbusa* in the prevention of HIV/AIDS and related subjects, in S. Mutonyi (ed), *Report of the 6th AIDS Conference, Hopes, challenges and responsibilities*, Zambia National AIDS Network, Lusaka: 45–47.

Mushingeh, C. Chama, W. and Mulikelela, D. (1990–91) 'An investigation of high-risk situations and environments and their potential role in the transmission of HIV in Zambia: the case of the Copperbelt and Luapula Provinces', unpublished report for the Population Council of Zambia

Mutepa, R. (1994) 'Gender and AIDS NGOs', Paper presented at the Gender and AIDS Workshop, Lusaka, 10–11 October, 1994.

Mutonyi, S. (ed) (1996) *Hopes, Challenges and Responsibilities*, Report of the 6th National AIDS Conference, Zambia National AIDS Newwork, Lusaka 17–19 June.

Mwale, G. and Burnard, P. (1992) *Women and AIDS in Rural Africa*, Aldershot: Avebury.

Mwanza, I. (ed) (1993) Proceedings of the SWAAZ/PANOS International Conference on AIDS for Anglophone African Media, Lusaka, 2–8 October 1992.

Mwila, M. and Chipeka, R. (1989) *The National Theatre Arts and Music Festival on AIDS in Zambia 1989*, unpublished report, Lusaka.

Mziray, J. (1998) 'Boys' views on sexuality, girls and pregnancies', in M. Rwebangira and R. Liljestrom (eds), *Haraka Haraka: Look Before You Leap*, Uppsala: Nordic African Institute.

NACP [National AIDS Control Programme, Tanzania] (1996) *HIV/AIDS/STD Surveillance, Report No. 10*, Dar es Salaam.

NACP [National AIDS Control Programme, Tanzania] (1997) *HIV/AIDS/STD Surveillance, Report No. 11*, Dar es Salaam.

NACP [National AIDS Control Programme, Tanzania] (1998a) Medium Term Plan, Dar es Salaam.

NACP [National AIDS Control Programme, Tanzania] (1998b) *HIV/AIDS/STD Surveillance, Report No 12*, Dar es Salaam.

NACP [National AIDS Control Programme, Tanzania] (1998c) Strategic Framework for the Medium Term Plan 1998–2002, Dar es Salaam.

NACP [National AIDS Control Programme, Tanzania] (1999) *HIV/AIDS/STD Surveillance, Report No 13*, Dar es Salaam.

NASTLP [Zambia National AIDS/STD/TB & Leprosy Programme] (1993) First Resource Mobilization Meeting for the Second Medium Term Plan of Zambia National AIDS/STD/TB and Leprosy Programme, 9–10 December 1993, Lusaka, Zambia.

NASTLP [Zambia National AIDS/STD/TB & Leprosy Programme] (1994) *Strategic Plan, 1994–1998, a time to act, a time to care*, Lusaka.

NASTLP [Zambia National AIDS/STD/TB & Leprosy Programme] (n.d.) Tables on 1994 surveillance survey data.

NASTLP [Zambia National AIDS/STD/TB & Leprosy Programme] and UNICEF (1996) *HIV.AIDS Bibliography, an annotated review of research on HIV/AIDS in Zambia*, Lusaka.

NASTLP [Zambia National AIDS/STD/TB & Leprosy Programme] (1997) 'Total AIDS and ARC cases reported 1984–July 1997'.

Ndeki, S., Klepp, K. and Mliga, G. (1994) 'Knowledge, perceived risk of AIDS and sexual behaviour among primary school children in two areas of Tanzania', *Health Education Research* 9, 1: 133–138.

Ng'weshemi, Ties Boerma, J., Pool, R., Barongo, L., Senkoro, K., Maswe, M., Isingo, R., Schapink, D., Nnko, S. and Borgdorff, M. (1996) 'Changes in male sexual behaviour in response to the AIDS epidemic: evidence from a cohort study in urban Tanzania', *AIDS* 10: 1415–1420.

Nnko, S. and Pool, R. (1997) 'Sexual discourse in the context of AIDS, dominant themes on adolescent sexuality among primary school pupils in Magu district, Tanzania (Lake Victoria)', *Health Transition Review* 7 suppl 3: 85–90.

Ntukula, M. (1994) 'The initiation rite', in Z. Tumbo-Masabo and R. Liljestrom (eds), *Chelewa, Chelewa, the Dilemma of Teenage Girls* Uppsala: The Scandinavian Institute of African Studies.

Nyamuryekung'e, K., Laukamm-Josten, U., Vuyloteke, B., Mbuya, C., Hammelmann, C., Outwater, A., Steen, R., Ocheng, D., Msauka, A. and Dallabetta, G. (1996) 'STD services for women at truck stops in Tanzania; evaluation of acceptable approaches', *East Africa Medical Journal* 74, 6: 343–347.

Oakley, P. *et al.* (1991) *Projects with People, the Practice of Participation in Rural Development*, Geneva: ILO.

Obbo, C. (1993) 'HIV transmission; men are the solution', *Population and Environment* 14, 3: 211–243.

O'Malley, J. (1996) Societal context and response', in J. Mann and D. Tarantola (eds), *AIDS and the World II, Global Dimensions, Social Roots and Responses*, Oxford: Oxford University Press.

Panos Institute (1992) *The Hidden Cost of AIDS, the Challenge of: HIV to Development*, London: Panos.

Parker, B. and Patterson, D. (1996) 'Sexually transmitted diseases as catalysts of HIV/AIDS in women', in L. Long and E. M. Ankrah (eds), *Women's experience with HIV/AIDS, an international perspective*, New York: Columbia University Press.

Parker, R. (1996) 'Empowerment, community mobilization and social change in the face of HIV/AIDS', *AIDS* 10 suppl 3: S27–S31.

Patton, C. (1985) *Sex and Germs, the Politics of AIDS*, Boston: South End Press.

Patton, C. (1993) '"With champagne and roses": women at risk from/in AIDS discourse', in C. Squire (ed), *Women and AIDS, Psychological Perspectives*, London: Sage.

Pearce, J. (2000) 'Development, NGOs and civil society', in J. Pearce (ed), *Development, NGOs and Civil Society*, Milton Keynes: Open University.

Pim, A. and Milligan, S. (1938) Report of the Commission Appointed to Enquire into the Financial and Economic Position of Northern Rhodesia, London: Colonial Office.

Piot, P. (1998) Address to the VIIth Conference on Women and AIDS, Dakar, Senegal, 14–17 December 1998. Online. Available HTTP: http://www.unaids/speeches/dakar98.html.

Pitts, M., Bowman, M. and McMaster, J. (1995) 'Reactions to repeated STD infections:

psychological aspects and gender issues in Zimbabwe', *Social Science and Medicine* 40, 9: 1299–1304.

Prins, G. (1980) *The Hidden Hippopotamus, Reappraisal in African History: the Early Colonial Experience in Western Zambia*, Cambridge: Cambridge University Press.

Puja, G. and Kassimoto, T. (1994) 'Girls in education – and pregnancy at school', in Z. Tumbo-Masabo and R. Liljestrom (eds), *Chelewa, Chelewa: The Dilemma of Teenage Girls*, Uppsala: Nordiska Afrikainstitutet.

Quigley, M., Munguti, K., Grosskurth, H., Todd, J., Mosha, F., Senkoro, K., Newell, J., Mayaud, P., ka-Gina, G., Klokke, A., Mabey, D., Gavyole, A. and Hayes, R. (1997) 'Sexual behaviour patterns and other risk factors for HIV infection in rural Tanzania: a case control study', *AIDS* 11: 237–248.

Raja, S. (1993) Progress Report, Muchinka Teen Centre for the prevention and control of HIV/AIDS among youth, Mansa District, Luapula Province, January–September 1993 (mimeo).

Ranger, T. (1965) 'The "Ethiopian" episode in Barotseland, 1900–1905' *Human Problems in Central Africa* 27: 26–41.

Reid, E. (1997) 'Placing women at the center of analysis', in G. Bond, J. Kreniske, I. Susser and J. Vincent (eds), *AIDS in Africa and the Caribbean*, Boulder, Colorado: Westview Press.

Reid, E. (n.d.) 'Other ways of doing things: the lessons of Cairo', Study Paper #4, UNDP, HIV and Development Programme. Online. Available HTTP:: http://www.undp.org/ hiv/Study/SP4.htm.

Reid, E. and Bailey, M. (1992) 'Young women: silence, susceptibility and the HIV epidemic', Issues Paper #12, UNDP, HIV and Development Programme. Online. Available HTTP: http://www.undp.issues.

Republic of Zambia (1997) Mid-term Review of the Second Medium Term Plan (MTP II) for the Prevention and Control of HIV/AIDS in Zambia, Lusaka.

Republic of Zambia, Provincial Planning Unit, Western Province (1995) Report on the Outreach Activities for the Women World Conference in Western Province, Mongu.

Rivers, K. and Aggleton, P. (1998) 'Men and the HIV epidemic', Gender and the HIV Epidemic. New York: UNDP HIV and Development Programme. Online. Available HTTP: http://www.undp.org/hiv/genderlist.htm.

Rivers, K. and Aggleton, P. (1999) 'Adolescent Sexuality, Gender and the HIV Epidemic', HIV and Development Programme, Gender and the HIV Epidemic, UNDP. Online. Available HTTP: http://www.undp.org/hiv/genderlist.htm.

Robinson, D. (1998) 'Rethinking the public sector: NGOs, public action networks and the promotion of community-based health care in Tanzania, Development Policy and Practice, Working Paper No. 38, Open University.

Rowlands, J. (1997) *Questioning Empowerment, Working With Women in Honduras*, Oxford: Oxfam.

Rugalema, G. (1999) *Adult Mortality as Entitlement Failure, AIDS and the Crisis of Rural Livelihoods in a Tanzanian Village*, PhD thesis, Institute of Social Studies, The Hague.

Rugumyamheto, A. (1998) 'Pregnancy is not the end of education', in M. Rwebangira and R. Liljestrom (eds), *Haraka Haraka... Look Before You Leap*, Uppsala: Nordic African Institute.

Rwebangira, M. and Liljestrom, R. (eds) (1998) *Haraka Haraka... Look Before You Leap*, Uppsala: Nordic African Institute.

Rweyemamu, C. (1999) 'Sexual behaviouir in Tanzania'. in M. Foreman (ed), *AIDS and Men, taking risks or taking responsibility*? London: Panoz/Zed.

Sadik, N. (1994) The State of the World Population 1994: choices and responsibilities, New York, United Nations Population Fund.

Sandala, L., Lurie, P., Sunkutu, M., Chani, E., Hudes, E. and Hearst, N. (1995) '"Dry sex" and HIV infection among women attending a sexually transmitted disease clinic in Lusaka, Zambia', *AIDS* 9 suppl: 561–568.

Sanders, D. and Sambo, A. (1991) 'AIDS in Africa: the implications of economic recession and structural adjustment', *Health Policy and Planning* 6, 2: 157–165.

Santana, S. (1997) 'AIDS prevention, treatment and care in Cuba', in G. Bond, J. Kreniske, I. Susser and J. Vincent (eds), *AIDS in Africa and the Caribbean*, Boulder, Colorado: Westview Press.

Scheinman, D. and Mberesero, F. (1999) 'The Tanga AIDS Working Group: A partnership between traditional healers and biomedical personnel'. Paper presented at the First International Conference on Traditional Medicine and HIV/AIDS, Dakar, Senegal, 11–12 March 1999.

Schoepf, B. G., Walu, E., Rukarangira, W. N., Payanzo, N. and Schoepf, C. (1991) 'Gender, power and risk of AIDS in Zaire', in M. Turshen (ed), *Women and Health in Africa*, Trenton N.J.: Africa World Press.

Schoepf, B. G. (1992) 'Women at risk; case studies from Zaire', in G. Herdt and S. Lindenbaum (eds), *The Time of AIDS*, London: Sage.

Schoepf, B. G. (1993a) 'AIDS action-research with women in Kinshasa, Zaire', *Social Science and Medicine* 37, 11: 1401–1413.

Schoepf, B. G. (1993b) 'The social epidemiology of women and AIDS in Africa', in M. Berer and S. Ray (eds), *Women and HIV/AIDS: an international resource book*, London: AHRTAG/Pandora Press.

Schoepf, B. G. (1997) 'AIDS, gender and sexuality during Africa's economic crisis' in G. Mikell (ed), *African Feminism*, Philadelphia: University of Pennsylvania Press.

Seeley, J., Kengeya-Kayonda, J. and Mulder, D. (1992) 'Community-based HIV/AIDS research – wither community participation? Unsolved problems in a research programme in rural Uganda', *Social Science and Medicine* 34, 10: 1089–1095.

Seidel, G. (1993) 'The competing discourses of HIV/AIDS in Sub-Saharan Africa: discourses of rights and empowerment Vs discourses of control and exclusion', *Social Science and Medicine* 36, 3: 175–194.

Seketeni, D., Kamuzaza, H. and Mwansa, E. (1995) 'Luapula Province poverty profiles, coping strategies and safety nets', Paper presented at the Poverty Reduction Workshop for Luapula Province, Mansa, 20–22 November.

Sen, G. and Grown, C. (1988) *Development, Crisis and Alternative Visions, Third World Women's Perspectives*, London: Earthscan.

Setel, P. (1996) 'AIDS as a paradox of manhood and development in Kilimanjaro, Tanzania' *Social Science and Medicine* 43, 8: 1169–1178.

Setel, P. (1997) 'AIDS prevention with local implementers – overcoming obstacles', *World Health Forum* 18, 2: 215–217.

Sherr, L. (1993) 'HIV testing in pregnancy', in C. Squire (ed), *Women and AIDS, Psychological Perspectives*, London: Sage.

Sherr, L. (1996) 'Tomorrow's era: gender, psychology and HIV infection', in L. Sherr, C. Hankins and L. Bennett (eds), *AIDS as a Gender Issue, Psychological Perspectives*, London: Taylor & Francis.

Shuma, M. and Liljestrom, R. (1998) 'The erosion of the matrilineal order of the Wamwera', in M. Rwebangira and R. Liljestrom (eds), *Haraka Haraka*: *Look Before You Leap*, Uppsala: Nordic African Institute.

Siame, Y. (1998) *Youth Alive Zambia, BCP Experience*, Ndola: Mission Press.

Sikwibele, A. (1996) 'Gender relations and the role of education in the fight against HIV/ AIDS in Kapulanga, Mongu' Paper presented at the Workshop on Gender and AIDS, Dar es Salaam, 20–24 August 1996.

Sikanyika, B. (1996) 'Role of traditional structures in HIV/AIDS education', in S. Mutonyi (ed), *Report of the 6th AIDS Conference, Hopes, challenges and responsibilities*, Zambia Naitonal AIDS Network, Lusaka.

Sinpisut, P., Chandeying, V., Skov, S. and Uahgowitchai, C. (1998) 'Perceptions and acceptability of the female condom [Femidom] amongst commercial sex workers in the Songkla province, Thailand', *International Journal of STD & AIDS* 9, 3:168–172.

Sumbwa, N. (1996) 'Traditionalism, democracy and political participation: the case of Western Province', unpublished paper.

Sunday News (Tanzania), 7 April 1986.

Susser, I. and Kreniske, J. (1997) 'Community organizing around HIV prevention in rural Puerto Rico', in G. Bond, J. Kreniske, I. Susser and J. Vincent (eds), *AIDS in Africa and the Caribbean*, Boulder, Colorado: Westview Press, (1997).

Tawil, O., O'Reilly, K., Coulibaly, I. M., Tiemele, A., Himmich, H., Boushaba, A., Pradeep, K. and Caraël, M. (1999) 'HIV prevention among vulnerable populations: outreach in the developing world', *AIDS* 13 suppl A: S239–S247.

Thomas, A. (1998) 'The Role of NGOs in Development Management: A Public Action Approach', Development Policy and Practice, Working Paper No. 40, Open University.

Tibaijuka, A. (1997) 'AIDS and economic welfare in peasant agriculture: case studies from Kagabiro Village, Kagera Region, Tanzania', *World Development* 25, 6: 963–975.

Times of Zambia (1985).

Trivedy, R. (1999) 'NGOs in a global future', *Development in Practice* 9, 5: 623–626.

Tumbo-Masabo, Z. (1994) 'Conclusions', in Z. Tumbo-Masabo and R. Liljestrom (eds), *Chelewa, Chelewa: The Dilemma of Teenage Girls*, Uppsala: Nordiska Afrikainstitutet.

Tumbo-Masabo, Z. (1998) 'Training by symbolism and imagery – the case of Wagogo and Wayao', in M. Rwebangira and R. Liljestrom (eds), *Haraka Haraka... Look Before You Leap*, Uppsala: Nordic African Institute.

Tumbo-Masabo, Z. and Liljestrom, R. (eds) (1994) *Chelewa, Chelewa: The Dilemma of Teenage Girls*, Uppsala: Nordiska Afrikainstitutet.

Turshen, M. and Twagiramariya, C. (1998) *What Women do in Wartime, Gender and Conflict in Africa*, London: Zed Books.

Ulin, P. (1992) 'African women and AIDS: negotiating behavioural change', *Social Science and Medicine* 34, 1: 63–73.

UN (1996) *HIV/AIDS and Human Rights, International Guidelines*, Second International Consultation on HIV/AIDS and Human Rights, Geneva, 23–25 September 1996, organised jointly by the Office of the UN High Commissioner for Human Rights and the Joint UN Programme on HIV/AIDS.

UNAIDS (1997) *Women and AIDS*, UNAIDS Best Practice Collection Online. Available HTTP: http://www.unaids.org.

UNAIDS (1998a) AIDS in Africa, Johannesburg, UNAIDS Fact Sheet. Online. Available HTTP: http://www.unaids.org/highband/fact/saepap98.html.

UNAIDS (1998b) *Gender and HIV/AIDS*, UNAIDS Technical Update. Online. Available HTTP: http://www.unaids.org.

UNAIDS (1998c) Report on the global HIV/AIDS epidemic, June 1998. Online. Available HTTP: http://www.unaids.org.

UNAIDS (1999a) AIDS – 5 years since ICPD: emerging issues and challenges for women, young people and infants', UNAIDS Discussion Document.Online. Available HTTP: http://www.unaids.org.

UNAIDS (1999b) 'Delegates call on UNAIDS to ensure a well-coordinated UIN response to HIV/AIDS' Press release, New York, 2 July 1999, Online. Available HTTP: http://www.unaids.org.

UNAIDS (1999c) Differences in HIV spread in four sub-Saharan African cities, summary of the multi-site study, UNAIDS Fact Sheet, Online. Available HTTP: http://www.u-naids.org/highband/fact/lusaka99.html.

UNAIDS (1999d) Integrating gender issues in the response to AIDS in Africa, UNAIDS Draft Technical Note, Online. Available HTTP: http://www.unaids.org/doc3/cpp/fn526.html.

UNAIDS (1999e) Meeting Statement on the Africa Partnership Against HIV/AIDS, 23–24th April 1999, Online. Available HTTP: http://www.unaids.org/UNAIDS/doc/london%2Doutcome.htm.

UNAIDS (1999f) The UNAIDS Report. Online. Available HTTP: http://www.unaids. org.

UNAIDS (1999g) *AIDS Epidemic Update: December 1999*, Online. Available HTTP: http://www.unaids.org.

UNAIDS (2000a) Press release accompanying the UN Security Council's discussion of AIDS in Africa on 10 January 2000 Online. Available HTTP: http://www.unaids.org.

UNAIDS (2000b) Report on the global HIV/AIDS epidemic, June 2000. Online. Available HTTP: http://www.unaids.org.

UNAIDS (2000c) Table of country-specific HIV/AIDS estimates and data, June 2000. Online. Available HTTP: http://www.unaids.org.

UNAIDS/WHO (2000a) Epidemiological Fact Sheet [United Republic of Tanzania] 2000 Update, June 2000. Online. Available HTTP: http://www.unaids.org.

UNAIDS/WHO (2000b) Epidemiological Fact Sheet [Zambia] 2000 Update, June 2000. Online. Available HTTP: http://www.unaids.org.

UNDP (1995) *Human Development Report, 1995*, New York: Oxford University Press.

UNDP (2000) *Human Development Report, 2000*, New York: Oxford University Press. Online. Available HTTP: http://www.undp.org.hdr2000.

van Damme, L. and Rosenberg, Z. (1999) 'Microbicides and barrier methods in HIV transmission', *AIDS* 13 suppl A: S85-S92.

Van Eeuwijk, B. and Mlangwa, S. (1997) 'Competing ideologies: adolescence, knowledge and silences in Dar es Salaam', in W. Harcourt (ed), *Power, Reproduction and Gender: the Intergenerational Transfer of Knowledge*, London: Zed Books.

Vos, T. (1994) 'Attitudes to sex and sexual behaviour in rural Matabeleland, Zimbabwe', *AIDS Care* 6, 2: 193–203.

WAMATA Newsletter January–March 1999.

Watney, S. (1988) 'The spectacle of AIDS', in D. Krimp (ed), *AIDS: Cultural Analysis, Cultural Activism*, Cambridge, Massachusetts: MIT Press.

Webb, D. (Central Board of Health [Zambia]/Unicef) (1997a) Adolescence, Sex and Fear, reproductive health services and young people in urban Zambia, Lusaka.

Webb, D. (1997b) *HIV and AIDS in Africa*, London: Pluto Press.

Weeks, J. (1988), 'Love in a cold climate', in P. Aggleton and H. Homans (eds), *Social Aspects of AIDS*, London: Falmer Press.

Weeks, J. (1993) 'AIDS and the regulation of sexuality', in V. Berridge and P. Strong (eds), *AIDS and Contemporary History*, Cambridge: Cambridge University Press.

Weiss, B. (1993) '"Buying her grave": money, movement and AIDS in North-West Tanzania', *Africa* 63, 1: 19–35.

Whelan, D. (1999) *Gender and HIV/AIDS: taking stock of research and programmes*, text written by D. Whelan, Unaids Best Practice Collection (UNAIDS/99/16E) Online. Available HTTP: http://www.unaids.org.

Whitehead, A. (1999) '"Lazy" men, time-use studies and rural development in Zambia' unpublished paper, Department of Anthropology, University of Sussex.

Wight, D. and Bernard, M. (1993) 'The limits to participant observation in HIV/AIDS research', *Practicing Anthropology* 15, 4: 66–69.

Williams, G. (1990) *From Fear to Hope: AIDS Care and Prevention at Chikankata*, London: Actionaid, in association with AMREF and World in Need.

Wilson, M. (1955) *Good Company*, Boston: Beacon Press

Wood, K., Maforah, F. and Jewkes, R. (1998) '"He forced me to love him": putting violence on adolescent sexual health agendas', *Social Science and Medicine* 47, 2: 233–242.

World Bank (1992) *Tanzania: AIDS Assessment and Planning Study*, Washington: World Bank.

World Bank (1997) The World Development Report 1997: The State in a Changing World, New York: Oxford University Press.

World Bank (1998) World Development Report, Knowledge for Development, 1998/99, New York: Oxford University Press.

World Bank (1999) *Intensifying Action against HIV/AIDS in Africa, responding to a development crisis*, Washington D.C.: The International Bank for Reconstruction and Development, Africa Region.

World Bank (2000) World Development Report 1999–2000: Entering the 21st Century Washington: Oxford University Press.

World Health Organisation (1995) Women and AIDS: an agenda for action, Geneva.

Young, K. (1993) *Planning Development with Women, Making a World of Difference*, London: Tavistock.

'Zambia National AIDS Council and Secretariat' [493] Health L. Online posting, Available e-mail: health-1@hivnet.ch; 21 March 2000.

Zambia National AIDS Network [ZNAN] (1997) *1997 Annual Report*, Lusaka.

Zivi, K. (1998) 'Constituting the "clean and proper" body', in N. Roth and K. Hogan (eds), *Gendered Epidemic*, London: Routledge.

Index